Fasting for the Mind, Body, and Soul

A Guide to Ramadan Fasting

Maah Khan

Table of Content

Introduction to Ramadan Fasting

Ramadan Fasting is an important and deeply spiritual practice observed by Muslims around the world. This month-long practice involves abstaining from food, drink, and other physical needs during the daylight hours, and instead focusing on prayer, charity, and spiritual reflection.

Ramadan fasting is a significant religious practice observed by millions of Muslims worldwide. It is the ninth month of the Islamic lunar calendar and is considered a time of deep spiritual reflection, self-discipline, and increased devotion. During Ramadan, Muslims fast from dawn to sunset, abstaining from food, drink, smoking, and other physical needs.

Ramadan is a significant month in the Islamic calendar that involves fasting, increased prayer, and acts of charity. It is a time for self-reflection, spiritual growth, and strengthening one's relationship with Allah.

Muslims believe that by abstaining from food and drink during the daylight hours, they can develop greater self-discipline and empathy for those who are less fortunate.

While the physical and mental benefits of fasting during Ramadan are well documented, the spiritual rewards are equally important for Muslims. By performing good deeds, engaging in charitable acts, and increasing their worship, Muslims hope to attain greater closeness to Allah and earn His forgiveness and mercy.

Physically, Ramadan fasting can have several benefits:

1. Improved self-control and discipline: Fasting teaches self-restraint and discipline over physical desires. It helps individuals develop better control over their eating habits and encourages moderation in their daily lives.

2. Detoxification and cleansing: The body undergoes a natural detoxification process during fasting, allowing the digestive system to rest and reset. This can result in improved digestion and a sense of rejuvenation.

3. Weight management: Fasting can aid in weight loss and weight management as it limits the number of calories

consumed within a specified time frame.
However, it is important to maintain a
balanced diet during non-fasting hours.

Mentally, Ramadan fasting can have several
benefits:

1. Increased mindfulness: Fasting
    encourages individuals to be more
    mindful of their actions, thoughts, and
    behaviors. It promotes a heightened
    sense of awareness and reflection,
    allowing for introspection and personal
    growth.

2. Improved focus and clarity: With a
    disciplined routine and reduced intake of
    food, the mind can experience
    increased focus and clarity. This can be
    conducive to productivity and
    concentration in various aspects of life.

3. Empathy and gratitude: Fasting can
    foster empathy and compassion for
    those who are less fortunate. It provides
    an opportunity to reflect on blessings,
    cultivate gratitude, and engage in
    charitable acts.

Spiritually, Ramadan fasting holds immense significance:

1. Deepening of faith: Fasting during Ramadan is a fundamental pillar of Islamic faith. It allows Muslims to strengthen their connection with Allah, seek forgiveness, and deepen their spiritual devotion.

2. Self-reflection and self-improvement: Ramadan offers a period for introspection and self-evaluation. Muslims use this time to reflect on their actions, seek personal growth, and strive to become better individuals morally and spiritually.

3. Increased acts of worship: Ramadan encourages increased engagement in acts of worship such as prayer, recitation of the Quran, and charitable deeds. Muslims seek to enhance their spiritual connection and draw closer to Allah during this holy month.

It's important to note that while fasting offers numerous benefits, it may not be suitable for everyone. Individuals with certain health conditions, such as diabetes or pregnancy, should consult their healthcare providers before participating in fasting. It is essential to prioritize one's health and well-being while observing religious practices.

Ramadan fasting is a sacred and transformative practice that encompasses physical, mental, and spiritual dimensions. It serves as a time of self-reflection, increased devotion, and personal growth for Muslims around the world.

In this book, readers will learn about the history and significance of Ramadan Fasting, as well as the rituals and practices that are associated with it. They will gain a deeper understanding of the spiritual and physical benefits of fasting, and learn how to prepare themselves for the month of Ramadan.

This book also provides practical guidance for those who wish to observe Ramadan Fasting, including tips on meal planning, managing hunger and thirst, and staying focused on prayer and reflection.

Through clear and accessible writing, readers will come away with a deeper understanding of this important practice, and be inspired to embrace the spiritual benefits of Ramadan Fasting in their own lives.

Maah

Chapter 1

The Importance and Benefits of Fasting

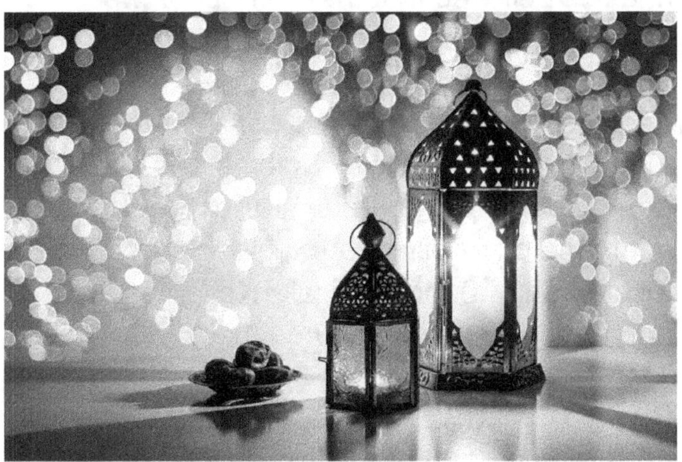

The history and significance of Ramadan fasting

Ramadan is the ninth month of the Islamic lunar calendar and is observed by Muslims worldwide as a month of fasting, prayer, and reflection. The practice of Ramadan fasting has deep historical and religious significance within Islam.

The origins of Ramadan fasting can be traced back to the revelation of the Qur'an, the holy book of Islam, to the Prophet Muhammad in the early 7th century.

According to Islamic tradition, the first verses of the Qur'an were revealed to the Prophet Muhammad during the month of Ramadan, and it is believed that the entire book was revealed to him over a period of 23 years.

Fasting during Ramadan is considered one of the Five Pillars of Islam, which are the basic acts of worship that are central to the Islamic faith. The other pillars are the declaration of faith (shahada), prayer (salat), charity (zakat), and the pilgrimage to Mecca (hajj).

During Ramadan, Muslims abstain from food, drink, and other physical needs from dawn until sunset. This includes abstaining from smoking, sex, and other activities that are considered worldly pleasures.

The fast is broken at sunset with a meal called iftar, which typically includes dates and water, followed by a larger meal.

The significance of Ramadan fasting goes beyond simply abstaining from food and drink. It is also a time for spiritual reflection, self-discipline, and charity.

Muslims are encouraged to increase their acts of worship and good deeds during Ramadan, such as reading the Qur'an, performing extra prayers, and giving to charity.

Ramadan fasting is also a time for communal celebration and togetherness. Families and friends often gather to break the fast and share meals, and mosques and other Islamic centers may hold special prayers and events throughout the month.

The history and significance of Ramadan fasting are deeply rooted in Islamic tradition and are an important aspect of the faith.

The month of Ramadan is a time for spiritual reflection, self-discipline, and community, and is a reminder of the importance of compassion, generosity, and humility in the Islamic faith.

What is Ramadan?

Ramadan is the ninth month of the Islamic calendar, and it is considered one of the most sacred months for Muslims worldwide. It is observed by Muslims worldwide as a month of fasting, prayer, and reflection.

During Ramadan, Muslims abstain from food, drink, and other physical needs during the daylight hours. They are also encouraged to avoid negative thoughts and behaviors, and instead, focus on spiritual purification, prayer, and acts of charity.

The fast begins at dawn and ends at sunset, and Muslims break their fast with an evening meal called iftar. The month of Ramadan ends with a celebration called Eid al-Fitr, which is marked by special prayers, feasting, and giving gifts to family and friends.

The evidence from the Qur'an consists of the following two verses: "O you who believe, fasting is prescribed for you as it was prescribed for the people before you in order for you to gain God consciousness, and,

"…The month of Ramadan, during which the Qur'an was revealed, a guidance for mankind, and clear proofs of the guidance and the criterion; and whoever of you is resident, let him fast the month" [al-Baqarah 185].

The Essential Elements of the Fast

The essential elements of the fast during the month of Ramadan, as observed by Muslims, include:

1. Intention: The fast begins with a sincere intention to fast for the sake of Allah.

2. Abstinence from food and drink: Muslims abstain from food, drink, and other physical needs such as smoking and sexual activity, from dawn until sunset.

3. Avoidance of sinful behavior: Fasting involves not only abstaining from food and drink but also avoiding sinful behavior, such as lying, backbiting, and engaging in other prohibited acts.

4. Increased prayer and worship: During Ramadan, Muslims increase their prayer and worship, particularly during the night-time prayers known as Taraweeh.

5. Charity: Muslims are encouraged to give to charity during Ramadan, as a way of showing gratitude to Allah and helping those in need.

6. Reading and reflecting on the Quran:
    Ramadan is a time for increased
    reflection on the teachings of the Quran,
    the holy book of Islam. Muslims are
    encouraged to read and study the
    Quran, and to reflect on its teachings.

7. Breaking the fast with dates and water:
    The fast is broken at sunset with dates
    and water, following the example of the
    Prophet Muhammad.

These essential elements of the fast help
Muslims to develop self-discipline, spiritual
awareness, and a sense of solidarity with those
who are less fortunate.

When Is Ramadan?

Ramadan occurs during the ninth month of the
twelve-month Islamic calendar, which follows
the phases of the moon.

This calendar doesn't align with the Gregorian
calendar used by much of the world, so
observance of this holy period doesn't start or
end on the same day each year.

In fact, it begins 11 days earlier every Gregorian calendar year and eventually passes through all calendar months over time. Ramadan 2022 begins on Saturday, April 2nd and ends on Monday, May 2.

Moon Sighting and Calculations for the start of Ramadan

The start of Ramadan is determined by the sighting of the crescent moon (hilal) of the ninth Islamic month. In Islamic tradition, the sighting of the moon is traditionally done by trained observers using naked eye.

However, in modern times, astronomical calculations have also been used to predict the appearance of the moon, and this method is considered valid by some scholars.

In recent years, many Muslim countries have adopted a combination of moon sighting and astronomical calculations to determine the start of Ramadan.

It is important to note that there can be differences in moon sightings and calculation methods between different regions and communities, and the start of Ramadan can vary accordingly.

Muslims should follow the guidance of their local Islamic authorities and scholars on the start of Ramadan.

The start of Ramadan is traditionally determined by the sighting of the crescent moon, but in modern times, astronomical calculations have also been used to predict the appearance of the moon.

Muslims should follow the guidance of their local Islamic authorities and scholars on the start of Ramadan.

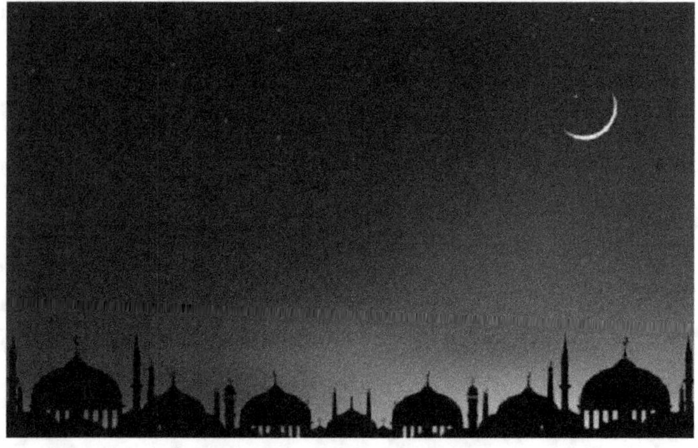

Should the New Moon for Ramadan Be Sighted or Calculated?

The issue of whether the new moon for Ramadan should be sighted or calculated is a matter of scholarly debate within the Muslim community.

Some scholars argue that the sighting of the crescent moon is the only acceptable method of determining the start of Ramadan as it is based on the Quran and the Prophet Muhammad's (peace be upon him) teachings.

They believe that relying solely on astronomical calculations can lead to inaccuracies and should not be used as the primary method of determining the start of Ramadan.

On the other hand, other scholars argue that advancements in astronomical technology have made it possible to accurately predict the appearance of the moon and that using astronomical calculations can provide a more reliable and consistent method of determining the start of Ramadan.

Ultimately, the decision on whether to rely on moon sighting or astronomical calculations for determining the start of Ramadan is up to the local Islamic authorities and scholars in each region.

It is important for Muslims to follow the guidance of their local Islamic authorities and scholars on this matter.

According to Sheikh Ahmad Kutty who is a Senior Lecturer and an Islamic Scholar at the Islamic Institute of Toronto, Ontario, Canada

1- During the time of Prophet Muhammad (peace be upon him), sighting the new moon with the naked eyes was the only means available for the people, as he himself said: **"We are a people who are unlettered."**

He did not mean that he would like his people to stay at that level forever. Given the condition of his time, the naked-eye sighting was the only possible choice.

2- We know from evidence that the Prophet used every opportunity to lift the Ummah out of illiteracy to literacy and civilization.

3- The Quran provides ample evidence for scientific observation of the sun and the moon. Astronomy today is a science that is based on observation of the position of the sun and the moon.

So, by following scientific methods of calculations, we are still observing the moon but not by naked eyes, rather by far more precise instruments.

Therefore, we are not contradicting the original intent of the Prophetic dictum that orders us to observe the moon.

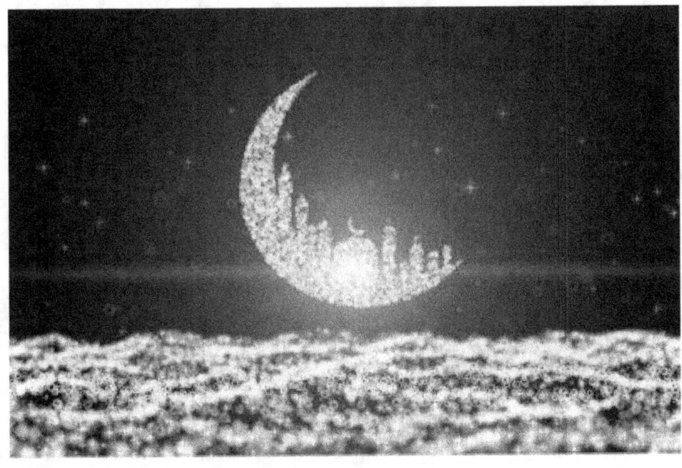

4- The fact that the scholars of the past did not base the beginnings of months on scientific calculations cannot be used as an argument, for in their time, there was little difference between astrology and astronomy.

Today, astronomy is a science. The Quran already taught us that the sun and moon revolve in their own orbits and that they follow fixed divine laws.

They do not run erratically, so there is an observable pattern to be discovered through observation, which is what scientists do.

That is why Imam Subki and others also supported calculations even before the snowballing of scientific knowledge.

Furthermore, by following calculations we can facilitate the observance of the festivals and plan for them way before their time. This is a great maslahah (public interest) for those living in the West.

The principle of taysir (facilitation) is a great consideration that we can never dispense with in this time and age.

What are the benefits of fasting in Ramadan

Fasting during Ramadan can have several benefits for individuals, including:

1. Physical benefits: Fasting can improve physical health by promoting weight loss, regulating blood sugar levels, reducing blood pressure, improving cholesterol levels, and improving digestion.

2. Mental and emotional benefits: Fasting can help individuals develop greater self-discipline, self-control, and patience. It can also promote a sense of inner peace and tranquility, as individuals focus on their spiritual growth and reflection during the holy month.

3. Spiritual benefits: Fasting during Ramadan is considered a way to purify the soul and increase one's spirituality. It can help individuals develop a stronger connection with Allah (God), gain a greater understanding of the Quran and Islamic teachings, and increase their level of devotion to Islam.

4. Social benefits: Ramadan is a time of community, solidarity, and generosity. Fasting can encourage individuals to be more compassionate, empathetic, and charitable towards others, leading to stronger social ties and a greater sense of unity.

5. Lifestyle benefits: Fasting during Ramadan can encourage individuals to adopt healthier lifestyles, such as eating a balanced diet, getting regular exercise, and avoiding unhealthy habits like smoking and overeating.

Fasting during Ramadan can have numerous benefits for individuals in terms of physical, mental, emotional, spiritual, and social wellbeing.

Additional Benefits during the month of Ramadan including:

1. Spiritual purification: Fasting is considered a way to purify the soul and strengthen one's relationship with Allah (God). By abstaining from food and drink during daylight hours, Muslims aim to focus their attention on their spiritual

growth and to become more mindful of their actions.

2. Self-discipline: Fasting is a way for Muslims to develop self-discipline and control over their desires and temptations. By denying oneself food and drink, one learns to be patient, grateful, and more disciplined.

3. Empathy and compassion: Fasting provides an opportunity for Muslims to empathize with those who are less fortunate and may not have access to basic necessities like food and water. It encourages Muslims to be more compassionate towards others and to be generous with their resources.

4. Community and solidarity: Ramadan is a time when Muslims come together to break their fasts and share meals with family, friends, and neighbors. It fosters a sense of community and solidarity, as everyone shares in the same experience of fasting and worship.

5. Gratitude and thankfulness: Fasting is also a way for Muslims to express their

gratitude and thankfulness to Allah for the blessings in their lives. By abstaining from food and drink, they are reminded of the importance of being grateful for the basic necessities of life.

What are the scientific reason for fasting in Ramadan

While the primary reason for fasting in Ramadan is religious, there are also several scientific reasons why fasting can be beneficial for individuals. Some of these reasons include:

1. Improved insulin sensitivity: Fasting during Ramadan can improve insulin sensitivity, which can help regulate blood sugar levels and reduce the risk of type 2 diabetes.

2. Reduced inflammation: Fasting has been shown to reduce inflammation in the body, which can help prevent chronic diseases such as heart disease and cancer.

3. Increased production of human growth hormone (HGH): Fasting can increase the production of HGH, which is

important for maintaining muscle mass and bone density.

4. Improved cognitive function: Fasting has been shown to improve cognitive function and brain health, possibly due to increased production of brain-derived neurotrophic factor (BDNF).

5. Enhanced immune system function: Fasting can enhance immune system function by reducing oxidative stress and inflammation in the body.

6. Improved cardiovascular health: Fasting can improve cardiovascular health by reducing blood pressure, improving cholesterol levels, and reducing the risk of heart disease.

There is growing scientific evidence to suggest that fasting can have a range of health benefits, many of which are consistent with the observed benefits of fasting during Ramadan.

Chapter 2

What is the difference between Ramadan fasting and intermittent fasting

Ramadan fasting and intermittent fasting are similar in that they both involve abstaining from food and drink for a certain period of time. However, there are some differences between the two.

Ramadan fasting is an annual religious practice observed by Muslims during the holy month of Ramadan. It involves abstaining from food, drink, and other physical needs from dawn until sunset for the entire month.

The fast is broken at sunset with a meal called Iftar, and another pre-dawn meal called Suhoor is consumed before the fast begins again.

Intermittent fasting, on the other hand, is a dietary approach that involves cycling between periods of fasting and eating.

There are several different methods of intermittent fasting, but the most common involves restricting food intake to a certain window of time each day, such as an 8-hour feeding window and a 16-hour fasting period.

While both Ramadan fasting and intermittent fasting involve periods of abstaining from food and drink, the duration and frequency of the fasts differ.

 Additionally, intermittent fasting is typically done for health and weight loss benefits, while Ramadan fasting is done for religious reasons.

What is suhr and Iftar and what can you eat?

Suhoor is the pre-dawn meal that Muslims consume before starting their daily fast during the month of Ramadan.

It is typically eaten before dawn and is considered an important meal as it helps provide energy and sustenance for the long day of fasting ahead.

The meal usually consists of nutrient-rich foods like whole grains, proteins, and healthy fats, as well as fruits and vegetables.

Iftar, on the other hand, is the meal that Muslims consume to break their fast at sunset during the month of Ramadan. It is considered a joyous occasion and is often shared with family and friends.

The meal typically starts with dates and water, in accordance with the Sunnah (tradition of the Prophet Muhammad), and is followed by a variety of foods such as soups, salads, bread, rice, and meat dishes, as well as sweet treats and desserts.

During Ramadan, Muslims are encouraged to eat healthily and in moderation, avoiding overeating and wasting food. It is also recommended to drink plenty of water and to consume foods that are nutrient-dense and provide sustained energy throughout the day.

Fasting during Ramadan is not only a spiritual practice but also a means of practicing self-discipline and developing empathy for those who are less fortunate.

What can you eat during intermittent fasting?

During intermittent fasting, there are different methods and schedules that can be followed, and the type and quantity of food that can be consumed will depend on the specific approach being used. Here are some general guidelines on what you can eat during intermittent fasting:

1. Time-restricted feeding: In this method, you limit your daily eating window to a certain number of hours, such as 8 hours, and fast for the remaining 16 hours. During the eating

window, you can consume a balanced and healthy diet that includes whole foods such as fruits, vegetables, lean proteins, whole grains, and healthy fats.

2. Alternate-day fasting: In this method, you alternate between a day of normal eating and a day of fasting, where you consume no or minimal calories. On the days of normal eating, you can consume a balanced and healthy diet, similar to the time-restricted feeding approach.

3. Modified fasting: This method involves consuming a limited number of calories on fasting days, such as 500-600 calories. During the eating window, you can consume a balanced and healthy diet similar to the time-restricted feeding approach.

It's important to note that during intermittent fasting, it's recommended to avoid highly processed foods, sugary drinks, and snacks, as they can increase hunger and disrupt the fasting state.

It's also important to stay hydrated by drinking plenty of water, and to listen to your body's hunger signals and eat until you feel comfortably full.

Consulting a healthcare professional or a registered dietitian can also be helpful in determining the best approach to intermittent fasting for your individual needs and health goals.

What are the pros and cons of intermittent fasting?

Intermittent fasting has gained popularity in recent years, and there are potential benefits and drawbacks to consider before deciding to adopt this eating pattern. Here are some of the pros and cons of intermittent fasting:

Pros:

1. Weight loss: Intermittent fasting can help reduce calorie intake and promote weight loss, which can be beneficial for individuals with obesity or overweight.

2. Improved insulin sensitivity: Intermittent fasting can improve insulin sensitivity, which can help regulate blood sugar levels and reduce the risk of type 2 diabetes.

3. Reduced inflammation: Intermittent fasting can help reduce inflammation in the body, which is linked to various chronic diseases.

4. Improved brain function: Some studies suggest that intermittent fasting may improve cognitive function, memory, and focus.

5. Simplifies meal planning: Since you're eating fewer meals throughout the day, meal planning and preparation may become simpler and more convenient.

Cons:

1. Hunger and cravings: Intermittent fasting can cause hunger and cravings, which may make it difficult to stick to for some people.

2. Fatigue and weakness: Some people may experience fatigue and weakness during the fasting period, especially during the initial stages of adopting the eating pattern.

3. Disordered eating: Intermittent fasting
   may trigger disordered eating behaviors
   in some individuals, such as
   binge-eating or restrictive eating.

4. Not suitable for everyone: Intermittent
   fasting may not be suitable for
   individuals with certain medical
   conditions, such as diabetes, eating
   disorders, or pregnant and
   breastfeeding women.

5. Can lead to overeating: Some people
   may overeat during the eating window,
   which can negate the potential benefits
   of fasting.

It's important to consult a healthcare
professional or registered dietitian before
adopting intermittent fasting to determine if it's
appropriate for your individual needs and
health goals.

**What are the pros and cons of Ramadan
fasting?**

Ramadan fasting is an important religious
practice for Muslims, and there are potential
benefits and drawbacks to consider before

deciding to observe this fast. Here are some of the pros and cons of Ramadan fasting:

Pros:

1. Spiritual benefits: Ramadan fasting is primarily observed for spiritual reasons, as it is believed to increase one's piety, self-discipline, and spiritual connection with Allah.

2. Community spirit: Ramadan fasting is observed by Muslims all over the world, which creates a sense of community and solidarity among Muslims.

3. Improved health: Ramadan fasting can have potential health benefits, such as weight loss, improved insulin sensitivity, and reduced inflammation in the body.

4. Improved eating habits: Ramadan fasting encourages healthy eating habits, such as consuming balanced and nutritious meals, and avoiding overeating and snacking.

5. Increased empathy: Fasting can also increase empathy and compassion

towards those who are less fortunate and experiencing hunger.

Cons:

1. Hunger and thirst: Fasting for long hours can cause hunger, thirst, and fatigue, which can be challenging for some people, especially in hot climates.

2. Disruption of sleep and daily routine: Late-night prayers and early morning meals can disrupt sleep and daily routine, leading to fatigue and decreased productivity.

3. Dehydration: Fasting for long hours can lead to dehydration, especially in hot climates or during physical activity.

4. Gastrointestinal problems: Eating large meals during suhoor or iftar can lead to digestive problems, such as indigestion, bloating, and constipation.

5. Not suitable for everyone: Ramadan fasting may not be suitable for individuals with certain medical conditions, such as diabetes, pregnant

and breastfeeding women, and the elderly.

It's important to consult a healthcare professional or registered dietitian before observing Ramadan fasting, especially if you have a medical condition or are taking medication.

It's also important to listen to your body's needs and to break the fast if you experience severe hunger, thirst, or any other health problems.

Which foods to break fast with?

The meal that is eaten to break the fast during Ramadan is known as Iftar. Muslims usually break their fast with dates and water, following the Sunnah (tradition) of Prophet Muhammad.

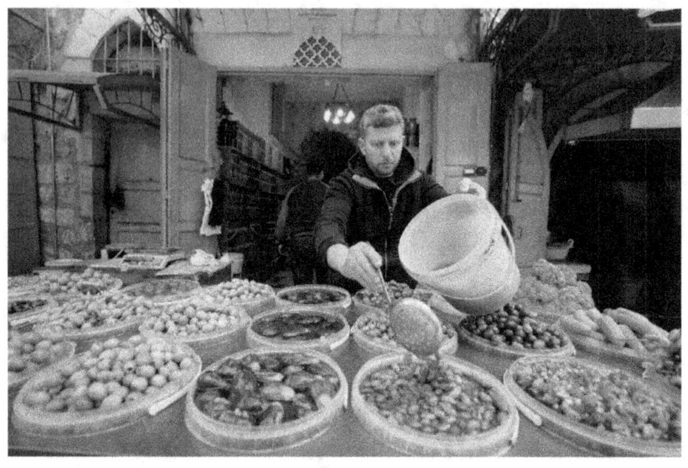

Dates are a rich source of natural sugars, fiber, and various vitamins and minerals, making them an ideal food to break the fast. However, there are many other foods that can also be eaten to break the fast, including:

1. Water: Drinking water is essential to stay hydrated after a day of fasting, and it helps to prevent dehydration during the night.

2. Fruit juices: Freshly squeezed fruit juices, such as orange juice or pomegranate juice, provide a good source of vitamins and minerals.

3. Milk-based drinks: Milk-based drinks, such as lassi or smoothies, provide a source of protein and calcium.

4. Soups: Light soups, such as lentil soup or chicken noodle soup, are a good source of nutrients and hydration.

5. Dates: As mentioned earlier, dates are a traditional food to break the fast, and they provide an immediate source of energy to the body.

6. Fresh fruits: Eating fresh fruits, such as bananas, apples, and grapes, provides a source of natural sugars, fiber, and vitamins.

7. Breads and grains: Whole-grain bread, rice, and other grains provide a source of carbohydrates, which provide energy to the body.

It is important to eat a balanced meal during Iftar, with a mix of carbohydrates, proteins, and healthy fats, to provide the body with the energy it needs to sustain itself until the next day's fast.

It is also important to avoid overeating and to eat slowly, to allow the digestive system to adjust after a day of fasting.

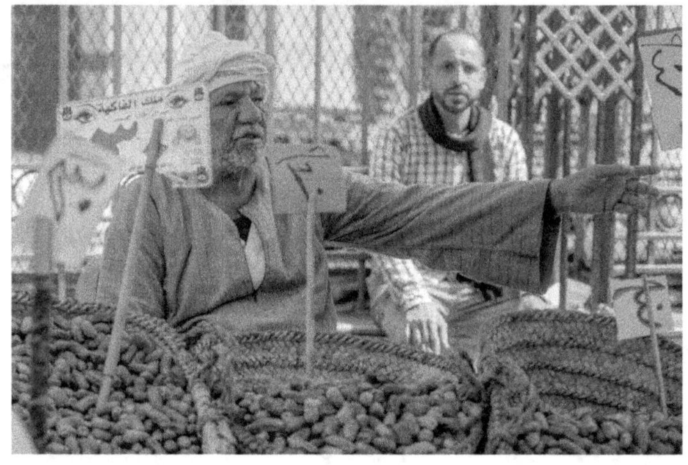

Chapter 3

How Does Fasting Affect the Human Body?

Millions of Muslims mark the month of Ramadan by fasting from sunrise to sunset each day. But what effects do those fasts have on the human body?

The month of Ramadan is a time of fasting and prayer for an estimated 8 million American Muslims and 1.6 billion Muslims worldwide.

For thirty days, observers forgo both food and water from dawn until dusk, only breaking their fast once the sun has set.

The practice of fasting isn't unique to Islam. For Hindus and Jains, single-day fasts mark auspicious occasions. Over the forty days of Lent, Christians undertake a partial fast. On the night before Yom Kippur each year, Jews begin a 25-hour period of fasting and prayer. Mormons are encouraged to fast for a day each month.

For most faiths, the sacrifice of food and water -- for hours, days, or weeks at a time -- is understood to be an intensely spiritual practice that allows for reflection and asceticism.

But while the spiritual importance of fasting is widely known, its physical effects on the body are less clear. How does the human body begin to change when it is systematically deprived of food and water, particularly over the long, hot, summer days of this year's Ramadan? Are there any biological benefits that accompany spiritual ones? Here are some answers.

Heart Health and Diabetes Prevention

A 2008 study conducted in Utah found that people who fast on a regular basis lower their risk of contracting coronary disease. In 2014, a follow up study found that fasting instigates metabolic changes and lowers "bad" cholesterol levels, which in turn can reduce the chance of heart disease by as much as 58%. That study also showed a decrease in blood sugar levels among people who fast.

Weight Loss

According to nutritionist Adam Brown, "Fasting should never be undertaken to lose weight. At the same time, some weight loss is reported by most people who fast." Once the body has used up its reserves of glucose, it burns fat for energy, which can result in some weight loss. Nutritionists warn, however, that excess fasting can lead to starvation and should be avoided at all costs.

Detoxification and Cleansing

Adherents of alternative food movements and medicine often undertake partial fasts during which they only consume vegetable juices. Proponents of juice fasts believe that they allow the body to cleanse itself of toxins absorbed from processed and fast foods.

Mental Health

Fasting may be religiously-mandated, but the social and communal traditions that accompany the practice carry just as much benefit. During Ramadan, families sit down to break their fast each night together. They visit relatives' and friends' homes for the nightly ritual, known as iftar.

The communal aspect of such fasting has been shown to impact the mental health of observers in a positive way. "Engaging in fasting can bring families and social groups closer together," said psychologist Susan Jones. "This often helps people suffering from depression and loneliness by reassuring them that they are not alone."

Breaking Addiction

Fasting, some say, gives the body time to pause and reset. That pause -- breaking from dietary routines -- can help to break food habits like sugar or caffeine addictions. Razia Ahmed, a student at New York University with a self-diagnosed "sweet tooth," says Ramadan helps her to break her chocolate-habit.
 "After Ramadan ends each year, it becomes much easier for me to control myself and stay away from the M&Ms," said Ahmed. "At least for a few weeks."

How Ramadan fasting effects the diabetics

Ramadan fasting can have significant effects on people with diabetes. During the fast, people with diabetes may experience changes in their blood sugar levels, which can have both short-term and long-term consequences.

For people with diabetes who choose to fast during Ramadan, it is important to consult with their healthcare provider to develop a plan for managing their diabetes during the fast. Here are some tips on how to manage diabetes during Ramadan:

1. Monitor blood sugar levels: People with diabetes should monitor their blood sugar levels regularly during the fast. This can help them detect and manage any changes in their blood sugar levels.

2. Adjust medication: People with diabetes may need to adjust their medication during the fast. This may include adjusting the dosage of their medication, changing the timing of their medication, or switching to a different type of medication.

3. Stay hydrated: People with diabetes should drink plenty of water and other fluids during non-fasting hours to prevent dehydration. Dehydration can affect blood sugar levels and increase the risk of other health problems.

4. Choose healthy foods: People with diabetes should choose healthy foods during non-fasting hours. This may include foods that are low in

carbohydrates, high in fiber, and rich in nutrients.

5. Break the fast with care: People with diabetes should break the fast with care to avoid a sudden spike in blood sugar levels. This may include eating small meals, avoiding high-carbohydrate foods, and monitoring blood sugar levels after breaking the fast.

It is important for people with diabetes to talk to their healthcare provider before starting Ramadan fasting. With careful planning and management, people with diabetes can safely participate in Ramadan fasting and experience the spiritual benefits of this holy month.

How to eliminate sugar craving during fasting

Eliminating sugar cravings during fasting can be challenging, but there are several strategies that can help:

1. Drink plenty of water: Staying hydrated can help reduce cravings and keep you feeling full. Aim for at least 8 glasses of water per day.

2. Eat balanced meals: Make sure to include complex carbohydrates, healthy fats, and protein in your meals. This can help stabilize blood sugar levels and reduce cravings.

3. Choose nutrient-dense foods: Foods that are high in nutrients, such as fruits, vegetables, and whole grains, can help satisfy cravings and provide sustained energy.

4. Avoid processed foods: Processed foods, such as candy, soda, and baked goods, are often high in sugar and can increase cravings. Try to choose whole foods instead.

5. Incorporate healthy snacks: Snacks such as nuts, seeds, and fruit can help satisfy cravings and provide sustained energy throughout the day.

6. Get enough sleep: Lack of sleep can increase cravings and disrupt hormones that regulate hunger. Aim for 7-8 hours of sleep per night.

7. Manage stress: Stress can trigger cravings and make it difficult to resist unhealthy foods. Try relaxation techniques such as deep breathing, meditation, or yoga to reduce stress.

It's important to remember that occasional sugar cravings are normal and nothing to be ashamed of. However, if sugar cravings are persistent or interfering with your daily life, it may be helpful to consult with a healthcare provider or a registered dietitian for additional support.

What is leptin? How it helps with sugar craving

Leptin is a hormone produced by fat cells in the body that helps regulate appetite and energy balance. It plays a key role in signaling the brain to decrease hunger and increase energy expenditure when there is enough stored fat in the body.

Leptin helps with sugar cravings by regulating the reward pathways in the brain that are associated with food intake.

When leptin levels are high, the brain receives a signal to decrease food intake and reduce cravings for sugar and other high-calorie foods.

However, in some cases, leptin resistance can occur, which can lead to increased cravings for sugar and other high-calorie foods. Leptin resistance occurs when the brain becomes less responsive to leptin signals, which can occur due to factors such as high levels of inflammation, stress, or a diet high in processed and high-calorie foods.

To support healthy leptin levels and reduce sugar cravings, it is important to maintain a healthy diet, exercise regularly, manage stress, and get enough sleep.

Additionally, consuming foods that are high in fiber, protein, and healthy fats can help regulate blood sugar levels and support healthy leptin signaling.

Consult with a healthcare provider or a registered dietitian for personalized recommendations on how to support healthy leptin levels and manage sugar cravings.

How Ramadan fasting effects the blood pressure

Ramadan fasting can have both positive and negative effects on blood pressure. Some studies have shown that fasting during Ramadan may help to lower blood pressure, while others have shown that it can lead to temporary increases in blood pressure.

During the fast, the body undergoes changes that can affect blood pressure. For example, dehydration can cause the blood to become thicker and more difficult to pump, which can increase blood pressure. In addition, fasting can lead to changes in hormones that regulate blood pressure, such as renin and aldosterone.

However, some studies have also suggested that fasting during Ramadan can have long term benefits for blood pressure. One study found that people who fasted during Ramadan had lower blood pressure six months after the fast ended compared to those who did not fast.

It is important for people with high blood pressure to talk to their healthcare provider before starting Ramadan fasting. They may need to adjust their medication or monitor their blood pressure more closely during the fast.

Here are some tips for managing blood pressure during Ramadan:

1. Stay hydrated: Drink plenty of water and other fluids during non-fasting hours to prevent dehydration.

2. Avoid salty foods: Eating foods that are high in salt can increase blood pressure. Choose foods that are low in salt and avoid adding extra salt to your meals.

3. Take medication as prescribed: If you are taking medication for high blood pressure, take it as prescribed by your healthcare provider.

4. Monitor blood pressure regularly: People with high blood pressure should monitor their blood pressure regularly during the fast to detect any changes.

5. Break the fast with care: Avoid overeating and eating foods that are high in salt or sugar when breaking the

fast. This can help prevent sudden changes in blood pressure.

With careful management, people with high blood pressure can safely participate in Ramadan fasting and experience the spiritual benefits of this holy month.

How Ramadan fasting affects the human body's organs

Ramadan fasting can have various effects on the human body's organs. Here are some examples:

1. Digestive system: During Ramadan fasting, the digestive system gets a break from constant food intake, which can help reduce inflammation and promote gut health.

    However, when the body breaks down stored fats for energy, it produces ketones, which can lead to bad breath, constipation, and other digestive issues.

2. Liver: The liver plays a crucial role in regulating blood sugar levels during fasting. When the body is not receiving food, the liver releases stored glucose to

keep the body functioning. This can lead to changes in liver function and may affect people with liver disease.

3. Kidneys: The kidneys are responsible for filtering waste from the body, and fasting can put additional stress on them. In some cases, fasting can lead to dehydration, which can affect kidney function.

4. Heart: Fasting during Ramadan can have both positive and negative effects on heart health. Some studies have shown that fasting can help reduce blood pressure, improve cholesterol levels, and reduce inflammation.

5. However, fasting can also lead to dehydration and changes in blood sugar levels, which can put additional stress on the heart.

6. Brain: Fasting can affect brain function, particularly in the areas of memory and cognitive performance. Some studies have shown that fasting can improve brain function and protect against age-related cognitive decline.

It is important to note that the effects of Ramadan fasting on the body's organs can vary depending on factors such as age, health status, and the length and intensity of the fast.

If you have any concerns about the effects of fasting on your body, it is important to consult with your healthcare provider.

They can help you develop a plan for fasting that takes into account your individual health needs and concerns.

How fasting during Ramadan benefit your:

- **Brain function:**

  Fasting during Ramadan can have several potential benefits for brain function, including improved cognitive performance and increased neuroplasticity.

  Studies have shown that fasting can increase the production of brain-derived neurotrophic factor (BDNF), a protein that promotes the growth and survival of neurons in the brain.

This increase in BDNF production can lead to enhanced neuroplasticity, which is the brain's ability to adapt and change in response to new experiences.

Fasting can also improve cognitive function by increasing the production of hormones such as norepinephrine and dopamine, which can help improve focus, attention, and mood.

Furthermore, fasting has been shown to reduce oxidative stress and inflammation in the brain, which can help protect against neurodegenerative diseases such as Alzheimer's and Parkinson's.

However, it is important to note that these potential benefits of fasting on brain function are largely based on animal studies and more research is needed to confirm these effects in humans.

Additionally, it is important to maintain a balanced and nutritious diet during non-fasting hours to ensure that the brain is receiving adequate nutrients to function properly.

Fasting during Ramadan may offer potential benefits for brain function, but it is important to consult with a healthcare provider or a registered dietitian if you have any concerns about your health or diet during fasting periods.

- **Confidence: How fasting during Ramadan benefit your Confidence**

  Fasting during Ramadan can potentially benefit your confidence in several ways, particularly through the cultivation of self-discipline and spiritual reflection.

  Fasting requires self-discipline, as it involves abstaining from food and drink during daylight hours for a month. This discipline can help individuals develop a sense of self-control, which can translate to other areas of their lives, such as work, relationships, and personal goals. As individuals successfully complete the fast each day, they can experience a sense of accomplishment and self-confidence, which can help boost their overall confidence.

In addition to self-discipline, fasting during Ramadan also involves increased spiritual reflection and connection with one's faith. This can lead to a greater sense of purpose and meaning in life, which can contribute to a sense of confidence and wellbeing.

Moreover, during Ramadan, many people engage in charitable acts and community service, which can help increase feelings of self-worth and confidence by contributing to the greater good.

However, it is important to note that the benefits of fasting on confidence are subjective and may vary from person to person.

It is also important to maintain a balanced and healthy lifestyle during non-fasting hours to ensure that your body and mind are receiving the necessary nutrients and rest to function properly.

Fasting during Ramadan can potentially
benefit your confidence through the
cultivation of self-discipline, spiritual
reflection, and community service, but it
is important to consult with a healthcare
provider or a religious leader if you have
any concerns about your health or
religious obligations during fasting
periods.

- **Clarity: How fasting during Ramadan
  benefit your Clarity.**

Fasting during Ramadan can potentially
benefit your clarity in several ways,
particularly through the improvement of
cognitive function and emotional
wellbeing.

Fasting can improve cognitive function
by increasing the production of
hormones such as norepinephrine and
dopamine, which can help improve
focus, attention, and mood. Additionally,
fasting can reduce oxidative stress and
inflammation in the brain, which can

help protect against cognitive decline and improve overall brain health.

Furthermore, fasting during Ramadan involves increased spiritual reflection and connection with one's faith, which can lead to a greater sense of purpose and meaning in life. This can help individuals gain clarity in their personal goals, values, and priorities.

Additionally, fasting can also help individuals gain clarity in their eating habits and relationship with food.

By abstaining from food and drink during daylight hours, individuals can become more mindful of their eating habits and may develop a greater appreciation for the food they consume. This can help individuals make healthier choices and cultivate a more balanced and nutritious diet.

However, it is important to note that the benefits of fasting on clarity are subjective and may vary from person to person. It is also important to maintain a balanced and healthy lifestyle during non-fasting hours to ensure that your body and mind are receiving the necessary nutrients and rest to function properly.

Fasting during Ramadan can potentially benefit your clarity through the improvement of cognitive function, emotional wellbeing, and mindfulness of eating habits, but it is important to consult with a healthcare provider or a religious leader if you have any concerns about your health or religious obligations during fasting periods.

- **Clear skin:How fasting during Ramadan benefit your Clear skin**

Fasting during Ramadan can potentially benefit your skin health in several ways, particularly through the improvement of hydration and reduction of inflammation.

During fasting periods, individuals abstain from food and drink during daylight hours, which can help improve hydration levels in the body. This can potentially lead to improved skin hydration, resulting in a more moisturized and plump complexion.

Additionally, fasting can also reduce inflammation in the body, which can help alleviate certain skin conditions such as acne and eczema. This is because inflammation can exacerbate these skin conditions, and reducing inflammation can help improve the appearance and overall health of the skin.

Moreover, fasting during Ramadan often involves eating a more balanced and nutritious diet during non-fasting hours, which can provide the body with essential vitamins and minerals that are important for maintaining healthy skin.

However, it is important to note that the benefits of fasting on skin health are subjective and may vary from person to person. It is also important to maintain a balanced and healthy lifestyle during non-fasting hours to ensure that your body and skin are receiving the necessary nutrients and rest to function properly.

Fasting during Ramadan can potentially benefit your skin health through improved hydration, reduced inflammation, and a more balanced and nutritious diet, but it is important to consult with a healthcare provider or a dermatologist if you have any concerns about your skin health during fasting periods.

- **Better sleep:How fasting during Ramadan benefit your better sleep**

Fasting during Ramadan can potentially benefit your sleep in several ways, particularly through the regulation of hormones and the improvement of sleep quality.

During fasting periods, individuals may experience changes in their hormone levels, including increased production of growth hormone and decreased production of cortisol. These hormonal changes can help regulate the body's internal clock and promote a more restful sleep.

Additionally, fasting can also improve sleep quality by roducing snoring and sleep apnea, which are common sleep disturbances. This is because fasting can reduce inflammation in the body, which can help alleviate these sleep disturbances.

Moreover, fasting during Ramadan often involves a more structured routine and increased spiritual reflection, which can help promote a more relaxed and peaceful state of mind. This can help reduce stress and anxiety, which are common contributors to sleep disturbances.

However, it is important to note that the benefits of fasting on sleep are subjective and may vary from person to person. It is also important to maintain a balanced and healthy lifestyle during non-fasting hours to ensure that your body and mind are receiving the necessary nutrients and rest to function properly.

Fasting during Ramadan can potentially benefit your sleep through the regulation of hormones, the reduction of inflammation and sleep disturbances, and the promotion of a more relaxed and peaceful state of mind, but it is important to consult with a healthcare provider or a religious leader if you have any concerns about your health or religious obligations during fasting periods.

- **Productivity: How fasting during Ramadan benefit your productivity**

Fasting during Ramadan can potentially benefit your productivity in several ways, particularly through the improvement of cognitive function, energy levels, and time management.

Fasting can improve cognitive function by increasing the production of hormones such as norepinephrine and dopamine, which can help improve focus, attention, and mood.

This can help individuals stay alert and focused during work or other productive activities. Additionally, fasting can also improve energy levels by reducing the fluctuations in blood sugar levels that can occur with frequent eating.

This can help individuals maintain a more consistent level of energy throughout the day, which can lead to improved productivity.

Moreover, fasting during Ramadan often involves a more structured routine, which can help individuals manage their time more effectively.

This is because fasting requires individuals to plan their meals and activities around specific times, which can help promote a more organized and disciplined approach to daily tasks.

Furthermore, fasting during Ramadan involves increased spiritual reflection and connection with one's faith, which can lead to a greater sense of purpose and motivation in life. This can help individuals stay motivated and focused on their goals, which can lead to improved productivity.

However, it is important to note that the benefits of fasting on productivity are subjective and may vary from person to person. It is also important to maintain a balanced and healthy lifestyle during non-fasting hours to ensure that your body and mind are receiving the necessary nutrients and rest to function properly.

Fasting during Ramadan can potentially benefit your productivity through the improvement of cognitive function, energy levels, time management, and motivation, but it is important to consult with a healthcare provider or a religious leader if you have any concerns about your health or religious obligations during fasting periods.

- Fat burning:Fasting during Ramadan can potentially benefit fat burning in several ways, particularly through the promotion of ketosis, increased metabolic rate, and improved insulin sensitivity.

- Ketosis is a metabolic state in which the body uses stored fat as its primary source of energy instead of glucose from carbohydrates.

During fasting, the body's glycogen stores are depleted, and it begins to rely on fat stores for energy, which can promote the production of ketones and the transition to a state of ketosis.

This can lead to increased fat burning and weight loss.

Moreover, fasting can also increase metabolic rate by stimulating the production of hormones such as growth hormone and adrenaline, which can help increase calorie expenditure and promote fat burning.

Additionally, fasting can improve insulin sensitivity, which is the ability of the body to respond to insulin and regulate blood sugar levels. Improved insulin sensitivity can help reduce the risk of insulin resistance and type 2 diabetes, which are associated with weight gain and difficulty burning fat.

However, it is important to note that the benefits of fasting on fat burning are subjective and may vary from person to person. It is also important to maintain a balanced and healthy lifestyle during non-fasting hours to ensure that your body and mind are receiving the necessary nutrients and rest to function properly.

Overall, fasting during Ramadan can potentially benefit fat burning through the promotion of ketosis, increased metabolic rate, and improved insulin sensitivity, but it is important to consult with a healthcare provider or a nutritionist if you have any concerns about your health or dietary needs during fasting periods.

- **Autophagy and fasting benefits**

Autophagy is a natural process by which cells break down and recycle damaged or dysfunctional cellular components, such as proteins, organelles, and other cellular debris.

Autophagy plays an important role in maintaining cellular health and preventing the buildup of damaged or toxic cellular components, which can lead to various diseases.

Fasting has been shown to stimulate autophagy in the body, which can have several health benefits. During fasting, the body's energy stores are depleted, and cells begin to rely on stored fat for energy.

This can lead to an increase in autophagy, as cells break down and recycle damaged cellular components for energy.

Some potential benefits of autophagy induced by fasting include:

1. Improved cellular function: By removing damaged cellular components, autophagy can help improve cellular function and prevent the buildup of toxic

cellular debris that can contribute to disease.

2. Reduced inflammation: Autophagy has been shown to reduce inflammation in the body, which is a key factor in the development of many chronic diseases.

3. Enhanced immune function: Autophagy can help enhance immune function by removing damaged or infected cells, which can help prevent the spread of infection and reduce the risk of developing autoimmune disorders.

4. Improved metabolic function: Autophagy has been shown to improve metabolic function and help regulate blood sugar levels, which can reduce the risk of developing type 2 diabetes.

It is important to note that the benefits of autophagy induced by fasting are still being studied, and more research is needed to fully understand the mechanisms behind these benefits.

Additionally, it is important to consult with a healthcare provider or a registered dietitian if you have any concerns about your health or dietary needs during fasting periods.

- **Anti aging and fasting benefits**

Fasting has been shown to have potential anti-aging benefits. Some of these benefits may be attributed to the process of autophagy, which occurs during fasting and helps to remove damaged or dysfunctional cellular components, which can lead to cellular rejuvenation and a reduction in the effects of aging.

Other potential anti-aging benefits of fasting include:

1. Improved insulin sensitivity: Fasting has been shown to improve insulin sensitivity, which is a key factor in age-related diseases such as type 2 diabetes.

2. Reduced inflammation: Chronic inflammation is a major contributor to many age-related diseases, including cardiovascular disease, Alzheimer's disease, and cancer. Fasting has been shown to reduce inflammation in the

body, which may help slow the aging process.

3. Increased production of growth hormone: Fasting has been shown to increase the production of growth hormone, which is important for cellular repair and regeneration.

4. Enhanced cellular repair: Fasting has been shown to enhance the body's natural cellular repair mechanisms, including DNA repair, which can help prevent age-related damage and disease.

5. Improved cognitive function: Fasting has been shown to improve cognitive function and protect against age-related cognitive decline.

It is important to note that the potential anti-aging benefits of fasting are still being studied, and more research is needed to fully understand the mechanisms behind these benefits.

Additionally, it is important to consult with a healthcare provider or a registered dietitian if you have any concerns about your health or dietary needs during fasting periods.

- **Longevity and fasting benefits**

Fasting has been studied for its potential benefits on longevity. Some studies have suggested that fasting may help to slow the aging process and increase lifespan by reducing oxidative stress, improving insulin sensitivity, and enhancing cellular repair mechanisms.

Here are some potential benefits of fasting on longevity:

1. Increased cellular repair: Fasting has been shown to enhance the body's natural cellular repair mechanisms, including DNA repair, which can help prevent age-related damage and disease.

2. Reduced oxidative stress: Oxidative stress is a key factor in the aging process, as it can damage cells and contribute to the development of age-related diseases. Fasting has been shown to reduce oxidative stress and improve cellular function.

3. Improved insulin sensitivity: Fasting has been shown to improve insulin sensitivity, which is important for preventing age-related diseases such as type 2 diabetes.

4. Enhanced immune function: Fasting has been shown to enhance immune function, which can help protect against infections and diseases that become more common as we age.

5. Increased production of growth hormone: Fasting has been shown to increase the production of growth hormone, which is important for cellular repair and regeneration.

It is important to note that the potential benefits of fasting on longevity are still being studied, and more research is needed to fully understand the mechanisms behind these benefits.

Additionally, it is important to consult with a healthcare provider or a registered dietitian if you have any concerns about your health or dietary needs during fasting periods.

Fasting Reduces Cancer Risk

There is some scientific evidence suggesting that fasting may help reduce the risk of cancer, although more research is needed to confirm this.

One study published in the journal Nature Communications in 2021 found that fasting for 72 hours (or three days) helped to protect against chemotherapy-induced DNA damage in mice.

The researchers suggested that this could be due to the body's natural response to fasting, which includes a reduction in insulin and glucose levels, as well as an increase in the production of ketones.

Other studies have suggested that fasting can help to improve markers of cellular health, such as reducing inflammation and oxidative stress, which are both linked to the development of cancer.

One study published in the journal Cancer Research in 2012 found that alternate-day fasting in mice helped to reduce the incidence of lymphoma and breast cancer.

However, it is important to note that fasting alone is not a cure for cancer, and more research is needed to fully understand its potential benefits and limitations.

If you are considering fasting as a way to reduce your cancer risk, it is important to talk to your doctor first and to follow a safe and healthy fasting regimen.

Fasting normalizes ghrelin levels

Yes, it is true that fasting can normalize ghrelin levels in the body. Ghrelin is a hormone that is responsible for regulating hunger and appetite in the body. Ghrelin levels tend to increase when the stomach is empty and decrease after eating.

During fasting, the body goes into a state of ketosis, which is a metabolic process where the body uses stored fat as its primary source of energy. This can lead to a decrease in the level of insulin in the body, which in turn can decrease the level of ghrelin.

Several studies have shown that fasting can lead to a decrease in ghrelin levels. For example, a study published in the journal Nutrients in 2019 found that intermittent fasting led to a decrease in ghrelin levels in overweight and obese adults.

However, it is important to note that the effects of fasting on ghrelin levels may vary depending on the type of fasting and the individual's overall health.

Fasting for too long or too frequently can also have negative effects on the body, such as dehydration, fatigue, and nutritional deficiencies. It is important to talk to a healthcare provider before starting any fasting regimen

Chapter 4

Hadith on Ramadan

Uthman ibn Abu Al-Aas narrated: "The Messenger of Allah (PBUH) said: 'Fasting is a shield from the Hellfire just like the shield of any of you in battle.'" (Sunan Ibn Majah, 1639)

Abu Huraira (RA) reported Allah's Messenger (PBUH) as saying: "Allah SWT the Exalted and Majestic said: Every act of the son of Adam is for him, except fasting. It is (exclusively) meant for Me, and I (alone) will reward it.

Fasting is a shield. When anyone of you is fasting on a day, he should neither indulge in obscene language nor raise the voice; or if anyone reviles him or tries to quarrel with him, he should say: I am a person fasting.

By Him, in Whose Hand is the life of Muhammad, the breath of the observer of fast is sweeter to Allah SWT on the Day of Judgment than the fragrance of musk.

The one who fasts has two (occasions) of joy, one when he breaks the fast he is glad with the breaking of (the fast) and one when he meets his Lord he is glad with his fast." (Sahih Muslim 1151)

The revelations from God to the Prophet Muhammad that would eventually be compiled as the Quran began during Ramadan in the year 610 CE, but the fast of Ramadan did not become a religious obligation for Muslims until the year 624 CE.

The obligation to fast is explained in the second chapter of the Quran:
"O ye who believe! Fasting is prescribed to you as it was prescribed to those before you, that ye may (learn) self-restraint…Ramadan is the (month) in which was sent down the Quran, as a guide to mankind, also clear (Signs) for guidance and judgment (between right and wrong). So every one of you who is present (at his home) during that month should spend it in fasting…" (Chapter 2, verses 183 and 185)

Anas ibn Malik reported: The Messenger of Allah, peace and blessings be upon him, said when the month of Ramadan began:
Verily, this month has presented itself to you. There is a night within it that is better than a thousand months. Whoever is deprived of it has been deprived of all good. None is

deprived of its good but that he is truly
deprived.

Source: Sunan Ibn Mājah 1644, Grade: Hasan
Abu Huraira reported: The Messenger of Allah,
peace and blessings be upon him, said when
the month of Ramadan arrived:

The month of Ramadan has come, a blessed
month in which Allah Almighty has obligated
you to fast. In it the gates of the heavens are
opened, the gates of Hellfire are closed, the
devils are chained, and in it is a night that is
better than a thousand months. Thus, whoever
is deprived of its good is truly deprived.
Source: Musnad Aḥmad 7148, Grade: Sahih
Greatness of Ramadan

Ibn Umar reported: The Messenger of Allah,
peace and blessings be upon him, said:
Islam is built upon five: to worship Allah and to
disbelieve in what is worshiped besides him, to
establish prayer, to give charity, to perform Hajj
pilgrimage to the house, and to fast the month
of Ramadan. Source: Ṣaḥīḥ al-Bukhārī 8,
Grade: Muttafaqun Alayhi

'Amr ibn Murrah reported: A man came to the
Messenger of Allah, peace and blessings be

upon him, and he said, "O Messenger of Allah, what do you think if I testify there is no God but Allah and you are the Messenger of Allah, I perform the five prayers, I pay the obligatory alms, I fast the month of Ramadan and stand for prayer in it. Among whom will I be?" The Prophet (ṣ) said: Among the truthful and the martyrs. (Source: Ṣaḥīḥ Ibn Ḥibbān 3492, Grade):

Below are 5 Ramadan Quotes from The Holy Quran.
"O you who have believed, decreed upon you is fasting as it was decreed upon those before you that you may become righteous" -- (Surat Al-Baqarah 2:183)

With the above verse, the Holy Quran makes it clear that fasting was ordained compulsory on all Muslims and that they have to fast if they are to stay righteous.
"...But to fast is best for you, if you only knew."
-- (Surat Al-Baqarah 2:184)

What the Holy Quran says about this blessed
month of Ramadan?

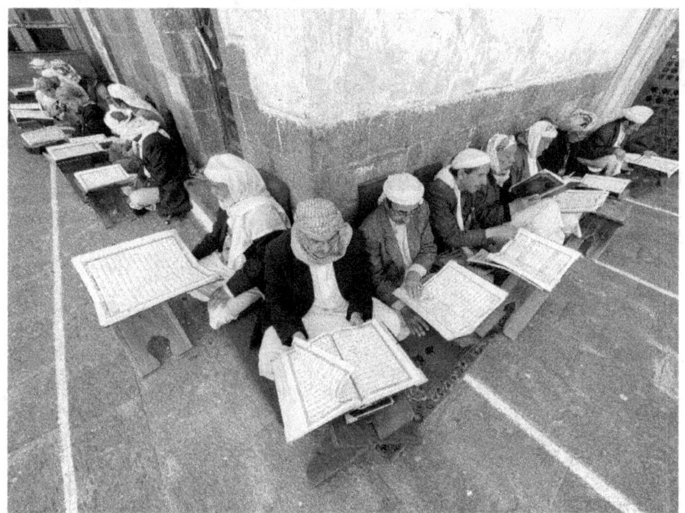

Quran says about Ramadan.Ramadan is an
important month in the Islamic calendar, and it
is mentioned in several places in the Quran.
Here are some verses that mention Ramadan:

1. "The month of Ramadan [is that] in
    which was revealed the Quran, a
    guidance for the people and clear proofs
    of guidance and criterion." (Surah
    Al-Baqarah 2:185)

2. "Ramadan is the month in which the
    Quran was revealed as guidance for
    mankind, clear proofs of the guidance,

and the criterion to distinguish right from wrong." (Surah Al-Baqarah 2: 186)

3. "O you who have believed, decreed upon you is fasting as it was decreed upon those before you that you may become righteous." (Surah Al-Baqarah 2:183)

4. "And eat and drink until the white thread of dawn becomes distinct to you from the black thread [of night]. Then complete the fast until the sunset." (Surah Al-Baqarah 2:187)

These verses highlight the importance of Ramadan as a month of fasting, reflection, and spiritual renewal. The Quran describes Ramadan as a time when the Quran was revealed as guidance for humanity, and it emphasizes the importance of fasting as a means of attaining righteousness and spiritual purification.

What Quran says about fasting

Fasting is an important act of worship in Islam and it is mentioned several times in the Quran. Here are some verses that mention fasting:

1. "O you who believe! Fasting is
   prescribed for you as it was prescribed
   for those before you, that you may attain
   Taqwa (piety)" (Surah Al-Baqarah 2:183)

2. "And those who give that (their charity)
   which they give (and also do other good
   deeds) with their hearts full of fear
   (whether their alms and charities have
   been accepted or not), because they are
   sure to return to their Lord (for
   reckoning)" (Surah Al-Mu'minun 23:60)

3. "O you who have believed, decreed
   upon you is fasting as it was decreed
   upon those before you that you may
   become righteous" (Surah Al-Baqarah
   2:183)

4. "The month of Ramadan [is that] in
   which was revealed the Quran, a
   guidance for the people and clear proofs
   of guidance and criterion." (Surah
   Al-Baqarah 2:185)

These verses emphasize the importance of
fasting as a means of attaining piety,
righteousness, and spiritual purification.

Fasting is prescribed not only for Muslims but for those who came before them as well. The Quran also highlights the spiritual benefits of giving charity during Ramadan and encourages believers to reflect on the Quran during this month.

Below are 5 Ramadan Quotes from The Holy Quran.
"O you who have believed, decreed upon you is fasting as it was decreed upon those before you that you may become righteous" -- Surat Al-Baqarah 2:183
With the above verse, the Holy Quran makes it clear that fasting was ordained compulsory on all Muslims and that they have to fast if they are to stay righteous.
"...But to fast is best for you, if you only knew."
-- (Surat Al-Baqarah 2:184)

In those days some might question the benefits of fasting apart from blessings. Science and medicine today have all but confirmed that there are numerous health benefits to fasting for a month in a year. It is a great way to cleanse the stomach and also has many health benefits for the brain.

"The month of Ramadhan [is that] in which was revealed the Qur'an, a guidance for the people and clear proofs of guidance and criterion. So whoever sights [the new moon of] the month, let him fast it; and whoever is ill or on a journey - then an equal number of other days.

Allah intends for you ease and does not intend for you hardship and [wants] for you to complete the period and to glorify Allah for that [to] which He has guided you; and perhaps you will be grateful." -- (Surat Al-Baqarah 2:185)

One of the stand out features of the month of Ramadan is that the Holy Quran was revealed to Prophet Mohammed (PBUH) during this time. This book of guidance is an invaluable treasure trove of information on how to live life as a good Muslim to this day.
"Allah is with those who restrain themselves." -- (Quran 16: 128)

Fasting teaches restraint; the ability to control worldly desires and spend time in prayer and meditation. Fasting is a noble act that is much beloved by Allah (SWT).

"Allah has made Laylat al-Qadr in this month, which is better than a thousand months, as

Allaah says...The Night of Al-Qadr is better than a thousand months.

Therein descend the angels and the Rooh [Jibreel (Gabriel)] by Allaah's Permission with all Decrees, there is peace until the appearance of dawn." -- (Al-Qadar 97:1-5)

The evidence from the Qur'an consists of the following two verses: "O you who believe, fasting is prescribed for you as it was prescribed for the people before you in order for you to gain God consciousness, and,

"...The month of Ramadan, during which the Qur'an was revealed, a guidance for mankind, and clear proofs of the guidance and the criterion; and whoever of you is resident, let him fast the month" [al-Baqarah 185].

Prophet practices of fasting

Fasting has been a practice in many religions, including Islam. Muslims follow the example of Prophet Muhammad (peace be upon him) who was known to fast regularly, not only during the month of Ramadan but also throughout the year.

The Prophet Muhammad (peace be upon him) would often fast on Mondays and Thursdays, and on certain days of the Islamic calendar, such as the 10th of Muharram (known as the Day of Ashura).

He also encouraged his companions to fast voluntarily as a way of drawing closer to God and increasing their spiritual growth.

During the month of Ramadan, the Prophet Muhammad (peace be upon him) would fast every day from dawn until sunset, and he would break his fast with dates and water, as was the custom at the time.

He would also offer the "tarawih" prayer at night, which is a special prayer performed during Ramadan.

Abu Huraira reported: The Messenger of Allah, peace and blessings be upon him, said, "When one of you hears the call to prayer while eating the pre-fasting meal and his vessel is in his hand, let him not put it down until he fulfills his needs from it."
Source: Sunan Abī Dāwūd 2350
Grade: Sahih (authentic) according to Al-Albani

Who were the first prophets to fast

 Abu Hurayrah that once the Prophet passed by a group of Jews in Madinah. The Prophet realized that they were fasting the " 10th day of Muharram ". The Prophet asked, " Why are you fasting this day? " They said this was the day when God rescued Prophet Moses and the Children of Israel from Pharaoh who drowned as well on that day.

It was also the day the ark of Prophet Noah landed on Mount al-Judiyy. Noah and Moses fasted that day as an indication of their thankfulness to God. Then the Prophet said, "I am the one to fast that day " and told his followers to fast the 10th of Muharram as well.

He justified the reason for fasting that day by saying, " We associate with Moses more than others do ". The Prophet said this because Moses was Muslim as all the prophets, and we are more deserving of rejoicing his victory.

Which days are forbidden to fast in Islam?

In Islam, there are certain days when it is forbidden to fast. These include:

1. Eid al-Fitr: This is the festival that marks the end of the month of Ramadan. It is forbidden to fast on this day as it is a day of celebration and feasting.

2. Eid al-Adha: This is the festival that marks the end of the annual pilgrimage to Mecca (Hajj). It is also a day of celebration and feasting, so fasting is forbidden on this day as well.

3. The three days of Tashreeq: These are the 11th, 12th, and 13th days of the Islamic month of Dhul-Hijjah, which immediately follow the day of sacrifice (Eid al-Adha). It is forbidden to fast on these days.

4. The day of Arafat: This is the 9th day of the Islamic month of Dhul-Hijjah, which is the day before Eid al-Adha. It is recommended to fast on this day for those who are not performing the pilgrimage, but it is forbidden for those who are performing the pilgrimage.

5. The day of Ashura: This is the 10th day of the Islamic month of Muharram. It is

recommended to fast on this day, but it is not forbidden to eat or drink if one chooses not to fast.

6. It is also forbidden to single out Fridays and only fast every Friday, as 'Abdullah b. 'Amr b. al-'As said that he heard Muhammad say "Verily, Friday is an eid (holiday) for you, so do not fast on it unless you fast the day before or after it."

7. Fasting every day of the year is considered non-rewarding; Muhammad said: "There is no reward for fasting for the one who perpetually fasts." This Hadith is considered authentic by Sunni scholars.

It is important to note that these are the only days on which fasting is forbidden in Islam. Muslims are encouraged to fast voluntarily throughout the year, outside of the month of Ramadan, as a way of increasing their spirituality and drawing closer to God.

Chapter 5

What age Ramadan fasting starts?

The age at which Ramadan fasting starts can vary depending on cultural and religious traditions.

In Islam, children are not required to fast until they have reached puberty and are considered to be adults in the eyes of the community.

However, some children may start fasting earlier as a way to practice and prepare for Ramadan fasting when they reach puberty.

It is important for parents to make sure that their children are physically and mentally ready to fast. Children who are too young or not yet ready to fast should not be forced to do so.

Instead, parents can encourage children to participate in other aspects of Ramadan, such as attending mosque, giving to charity, and performing good deeds.

As children reach puberty and become adults, they are expected to fast during Ramadan unless they have a health condition that prevents them from doing so.

In some cases, pregnant or breastfeeding women, people with certain medical conditions, and travelers may be exempt from fasting.

It is important for individuals to consult with their healthcare provider and religious leaders to determine if they are healthy enough to fast and if they are eligible for any exemptions.

Who are not allowed to fast in Ramadan?

While fasting during Ramadan is mandatory for most adult Muslims, there are some exceptions and circumstances under which individuals are not allowed to fast. These include:

1. Children who have not yet reached puberty: Children are not required to fast until they have reached puberty and are considered to be adults in the eyes of the community.

2. People who are ill or have a medical condition: Those who are ill or have a medical condition that makes fasting dangerous or harmful to their health are exempt from fasting.

3. This includes people with diabetes, heart disease, and other chronic conditions.

4. Pregnant and breastfeeding women: Women who are pregnant or breastfeeding may choose not to fast if they believe it will harm their health or the health of their baby.

5. Women during their menstrual cycle: Women who are menstruating are not allowed to fast during their period, but they must make up the missed days of fasting after their period ends.

6. Travelers: Muslims who are traveling long distances are allowed to break their fast and make up the missed days of fasting later.

It is important to note that individuals who are exempt from fasting are still expected to participate in other aspects of Ramadan, such as prayer, charitable giving, and acts of kindness and perform other good deeds as a way of participating in the spiritual and communal aspects of Ramadan.

What menstrual women can do during Ramadan?

Menstrual women are exempted from fasting during Ramadan as fasting is not obligatory during menstruation.

However, there are still several ways in which they can participate in the spiritual and social aspects of Ramadan. Here are some suggestions:

1. Recite Quran and engage in other forms of worship: Menstrual women can engage in other forms of worship during Ramadan, such as reciting Quran, making dua, and performing other voluntary acts of worship.

2. Give charity: Ramadan is a time for giving and charity, and menstrual women can participate in this by giving charity or helping those in need.

3. Attend Islamic lectures and gatherings: Many mosques and Islamic centers offer lectures and other gatherings during Ramadan. Menstrual women can attend these gatherings and benefit from the spiritual atmosphere.

4. Make up the missed fasts: After the completion of Ramadan, menstrual women can make up the missed fasts that they were exempted from due to their menstrual cycle.

5. Prepare iftar and participate in other social events: Menstrual women can prepare iftar (the meal that breaks the fast) for their family or friends, and participate in other social events during Ramadan.

In conclusion, menstrual women are exempted from fasting during Ramadan, but they can still participate in the spiritual and social aspects of Ramadan by engaging in other forms of worship, giving charity, attending Islamic lectures and gatherings, making up missed fasts, and participating in social events.

Things that can breach your fast in Ramadan

During the month of Ramadan, Muslims observe fasts from dawn until sunset. The purpose of the fast is to abstain from food, drink, and other physical needs during the daylight hours, in order to achieve greater self-discipline, patience, and spiritual purification.

Here are some things that can breach a person's fast in Ramadan:

1. Eating and drinking: Consuming any food or drink, including water, tea, and coffee, breaks the fast. Even if a person consumes a small amount unintentionally, the fast is considered broken.

2. Intentional vomiting: Vomiting intentionally, whether by sticking a finger down the throat or by consuming something that causes vomiting, breaks the fast.

3. Intentional swallowing of saliva: Although swallowing saliva is a natural process and cannot be avoided,

intentionally swallowing an excessive amount of saliva can break the fast.

4. Sexual intercourse: Sexual intercourse, even if it is done during the night, breaks the fast.

5. Menstruation and postnatal bleeding: Women who are menstruating or experiencing postnatal bleeding are exempt from fasting during this time.

6. Injections and blood transfusions: Any form of injection, including intravenous and intramuscular injections, breaks the fast. However, injections that are used for medical reasons are permissible, as long as they do not contain any nutrients.

7. Smoking: Smoking tobacco or any other substance breaks the fast.

8. If a woman gets her period anytime before sunset, her fast becomes invalid. Malik was asked what she should do about her fasting and prayer, and he said, "This blood is like menstrual blood. When she sees it, she should break her

fast, and then make up the days she has missed. Then, when the blood has completely stopped, she should do ghusl and fast." (Muwatta Malik Book 18, Hadith 49)

9. Moreover, in Sahih Al Bukhari 304, it says, "A woman can neither pray nor fast during her menses."

   It is important to note that if a person accidentally breaks their fast due to forgetfulness, they should continue fasting for the rest of the day, and their fast will still be valid.

   However, if a person intentionally breaks their fast, they must make up for that day of fasting at a later time or feed a needy person for each day missed.

What consider major sins during fasting in Ramadan?

During the month of Ramadan, Muslims are expected to observe fasting from dawn until sunset, and to engage in acts of worship and spiritual reflection. However, there are certain acts that are considered major sins during

Ramadan, which can nullify the rewards of fasting and may incur the wrath of Allah. Some of these major sins include:

1. **Intentional breaking of the fast:** Intentionally breaking the fast, such as by eating or drinking, without a valid reason is a major sin in Islam.

2. **Backbiting and slander:** Engaging in backbiting, slander, or spreading rumors about others is a major sin, and it is even more serious during Ramadan, when Muslims are expected to practice self-restraint and avoid negative behaviors.

3. **Engaging in sexual intercourse:** Sexual intercourse during the daytime, whether in or out of wedlock, is a major sin that breaks the fast.

4. **Neglecting the obligatory prayers:** Neglecting the five daily obligatory prayers or delaying them without a valid excuse is a major sin.

5. **Lying:** Deliberately lying or deceiving others is a major sin in Islam, and it

becomes even more serious during Ramadan.

6. **Engaging in sinful acts:** Engaging in any sinful act, such as stealing, cheating, or engaging in illicit behavior, is a major sin that can nullify the rewards of fasting.
7. **Fasting without a sincere intention:** Fasting without a sincere intention or for the sake of showoff is a major sin that can deprive a person of the rewards of fasting.

It is important to avoid committing these major sins during Ramadan, and to engage in acts of worship and spiritual reflection instead. By doing so, Muslims can achieve greater spiritual purification and draw closer to Allah.

How do you make up Ramadan missed fasts

If a Muslim is unable to observe the fast during the month of Ramadan due to illness, travel, or other valid reasons, they are required to make up the missed fasts at a later time. Here are the steps to make up Ramadan missed fasts:

1. Intention: As with any other fast, the intention to fast must be made before dawn.

2. Schedule: The missed fasts can be made up at any time throughout the year, but it is recommended to make them up as soon as possible after Ramadan.

3. Number of days: The number of missed fasts should be recorded, and one should make sure to fast an equal number of days.

4. Observance: One should observe the missed fasts in the same manner as the regular Ramadan fasts, by abstaining from food, drink, and other physical needs from dawn until sunset.

5. Intent: The intention for each missed fast should be made at the time of starting the fast.

6. Du'a: It is recommended to supplicate to Allah for His forgiveness and mercy.

It is important to note that for those who are unable to make up missed fasts due to chronic illness or other valid reasons, they can make a donation to feed a needy person for each missed fast instead.

Making up Ramadan missed fasts is an important aspect of the Islamic faith, and Muslims are encouraged to fulfill this obligation as soon as possible after Ramadan.

what happens if you can't make up missed Ramadan fasts?

If a Muslim is unable to make up missed Ramadan fasts due to a chronic illness, old age, or other valid reasons, such as being pregnant or breastfeeding, they can give Fidya or Kaffara instead.

Fidya is the compensation for missed fasts, and it involves feeding one needy person per missed fast. The amount of food given should be equivalent to what is normally eaten for one day, and it can be given all at once or in portions.

Kaffara is a penalty for intentionally breaking or invalidating a fast during Ramadan, and it involves either fasting for 60 consecutive days or feeding 60 needy people.

Kaffara is only required in certain cases, such as breaking a fast by eating or drinking intentionally, or engaging in sexual activity during the fasting hours.

It is important to note that Fidya and Kaffara are not substitutes for the missed fasts, but they are a means of fulfilling the obligation when one is unable to make up the missed fasts.

It is recommended to consult with a knowledgeable Islamic scholar or authority to determine the best course of action in individual cases.

Islam provides options for those who are unable to make up missed Ramadan fasts due to valid reasons, such as chronic illness or old age. Fidya and Kaffara are alternative means of fulfilling the obligation, but they are not substitutes for the missed fasts.

How Should I Make up for Years of Skipped Fasting?

If a Muslim has missed many years of fasting during Ramadan, they should make up for the missed fasts as soon as possible.

Making up for missed fasts requires commitment, dedication, and planning. Here are the steps to make up for years of skipped fasting:

1. Determine the number of missed fasts: The first step is to determine the number of missed fasts. This can be done by reviewing past years' calendars and counting the number of days missed.

2. Intention: One should make the intention to make up for the missed fasts with sincerity and dedication.

3. Plan and Schedule: One should plan and schedule the makeup fasts, making sure to spread them out over a reasonable period of time. It may be helpful to divide the missed fasts over several months or even years to make it more manageable.

4. Observance: One should observe the makeup fasts in the same manner as the regular Ramadan fasts, by abstaining from food, drink, and other physical needs from dawn until sunset.

5. Supplication and Du'a: It is recommended to supplicate to Allah for His forgiveness and mercy and to seek His help in fulfilling this obligation.

6. Fidya or Kaffara: If a Muslim is unable to make up missed fasts due to chronic illness or other valid reasons, they can give Fidya or Kaffara instead.

It is important to note that making up missed fasts is a serious obligation in Islam, and Muslims should strive to fulfill this obligation as soon as possible.

It may be challenging to make up for missed fasts from several years ago, but with dedication, planning, and supplication, it is achievable.

Making up missed fasts requires commitment and dedication. Muslims should determine the number of missed fasts, plan and schedule the makeup fasts, observe the fasts, supplicate to Allah for His forgiveness and mercy, and give Fidya or Kaffara if unable to make up the missed fasts.

There is,another view on this issue. This is a view held by Imam Ibn Taymiyyah. According to him, a person who had been away from Islam and now is repentant of his past sins and looks forward to leading a responsible Islamic life is not obligated to make up for the Prayers or fasts he or she has missed or neglected to do in the past.

Rather, it is enough for him or her to repent and ask Allah for forgiveness repeatedly.

The Prophet (peace and blessings be upon him) reassured us saying, "This religion of ours is simple and easy to comply with; so whoever makes it hard will only be defeated by it." (Al-Bukhari)

Chapter 6

Maintaining a Healthy Lifestyle During Ramadan

Tips on meal planning

Meal planning is an important aspect of observing Ramadan Fasting. Here are some tips to help you plan your meals during this holy month:

1. Plan your meals in advance: Before Ramadan begins, take some time to plan your meals for the month. This will help you avoid last-minute scrambling for food, and ensure that you have nutritious meals that will keep you energized throughout the day.

2. Eat a balanced diet: During Ramadan, it is important to eat a balanced diet that includes plenty of fruits, vegetables, whole grains, and lean protein. These foods will provide you with the necessary nutrients to keep you healthy and energized during the day.

3. Stay hydrated: It is important to drink plenty of water during non-fasting hours to avoid dehydration. Drink water and other hydrating fluids such as milk, coconut water, or fruit juice during the pre-dawn meal (suhoor) and after breaking the fast (iftar).

4. Avoid overeating: It is tempting to overeat during the evening meal, but this can lead to discomfort and sluggishness the next day. Instead, try to eat small, frequent meals throughout the night to help you stay energized and focused.

5. Choose healthy cooking methods: During Ramadan, opt for healthy cooking methods such as baking, grilling, or steaming instead of frying or cooking with heavy oils. This will help you maintain a balanced diet and avoid digestive discomfort.

6. Plan for leftovers: Plan your meals in a way that you can have leftovers for the next day's suhoor or iftar. This will save you time and energy in the kitchen and

ensure that you have nutritious food
readily available.

By following these tips, you can ensure that
you are eating healthy and balanced meals
during Ramadan, and that you are staying
energized and focused throughout the day..

Manage hunger and thirst:

Managing hunger and thirst during Ramadan
can be a challenge, especially if you are not
used to fasting.

1. **Start with a nutritious suhoor meal:**
    The pre-dawn meal (suhoor) is an
    important meal during Ramadan, as it
    provides you with the energy you need
    to get through the day.

    Make sure to eat a nutritious meal that
    includes complex carbohydrates,
    protein, and healthy fats. This will help
    keep you fuller for longer and prevent
    hunger pangs throughout the day.
2. **Stay hydrated:** It is important to drink
    plenty of fluids during non-fasting hours
    to avoid dehydration. Drink water and
    other hydrating fluids such as milk,

coconut water, or fruit juice during suhoor and iftar.

3. **Avoid caffeine and salty foods:** Caffeine and salty foods can cause dehydration, so it is best to avoid them during Ramadan. Instead, opt for hydrating fluids and foods such as water, fruits, and vegetables.

4. **Rest and conserve energy:** Resting and conserving energy during the day can help reduce feelings of hunger and thirst. Take breaks when needed, and avoid strenuous activities during the day.

5. **Keep busy:** Keeping busy can help distract you from feelings of hunger and thirst. Use this time to focus on spiritual reflection, prayer, or other activities that keep your mind engaged.

6. **Break your fast slowly:** When it is time to break your fast, start with a few dates and water before moving on to a full meal. This will help ease your digestive system into eating after a long day of fasting.

By following these tips, you can manage
hunger and thirst during Ramadan and
maintain your energy levels throughout the day.

Remember, fasting during Ramadan is an act
of devotion and spiritual reflection, so try to
focus on the spiritual benefits of fasting rather
than the physical challenges.
staying focused on prayer and reflection in
Ramadan is an important part of this holy
month.

Tips to help you stay focused:

1. **Create a schedule:** Creating a
   schedule for your daily activities can
   help you stay focused on prayer and
   reflection. Allocate specific times for
   prayer, Quran reading, and other
   spiritual activities.

2. **Disconnect from distractions:**
   Disconnecting from distractions such as
   social media, television, and other
   electronic devices can help you stay
   focused on your spiritual practices.
   Consider turning off your phone or
   computer during prayer times to avoid
   distractions.

3. **Find a quiet space**: Finding a quiet space where you can pray and reflect can help you stay focused. Consider creating a designated prayer area in your home where you can go to pray and reflect.

4. **Read the Quran:** Reading the Quran is an important part of Ramadan, and can help you stay focused on your spiritual practices. Consider setting aside time each day to read the Quran and reflect on its teachings.

5. **Attend Taraweeh prayers:** Taraweeh prayers are an additional prayer that is offered during Ramadan. Attending these prayers at your local mosque can help you stay focused on your spiritual practices and connect with other members of your community.

6. **Practice gratitude:** Practicing gratitude can help you stay focused on the blessings in your life and connect with your spirituality. Consider keeping a gratitude journal or taking time each day to reflect on what you are grateful for.

By following these tips, you can stay focused on prayer and reflection during Ramadan and connect with your spirituality on a deeper level.

Remember, Ramadan is a time of spiritual reflection, so try to make the most of this holy month and use it as an opportunity to connect with your faith.

Ramadan and workout

Ramadan is a month of spiritual reflection and devotion for Muslims, which includes fasting from dawn until sunset. Many Muslims who observe Ramadan may wonder whether it's possible to continue their regular workout routine during this time.

It is possible to exercise during Ramadan, but it's important to make some adjustments to your routine to ensure that you're able to maintain your energy levels and stay hydrated throughout the day.

Here are some tips for working out during Ramadan:

1. **Time your workouts appropriately:** Try to schedule your workouts for after Iftar or before Suhoor, when you're able to eat and drink normally.

   Avoid exercising during the hottest part of the day or immediately before breaking your fast, as this can lead to dehydration and fatigue.

2. **Adjust the intensity of your workouts:** During Ramadan, it's important to listen to your body and adjust the intensity of your workouts accordingly.

   Consider reducing the length or intensity of your workouts to conserve energy, or focus on low-impact activities like yoga or stretching.

3. **Stay hydrated:** Make sure to drink plenty of water and other fluids during non-fasting hours to stay hydrated.

During your workout, take frequent breaks to drink water and rest if you start to feel tired or lightheaded.

4. **Eat nutrient-rich foods**: When breaking your fast, prioritize nutrient-rich foods like whole grains, lean proteins, fruits, and vegetables to help replenish your energy levels and support muscle recovery.

5. **Consult with a healthcare professional:** If you have any medical conditions or concerns about exercising during Ramadan, it's important to consult with a healthcare professional before starting a new workout routine.

By making these adjustments to your workout routine, you can continue to stay active and healthy during Ramadan while still honoring your religious observances.

How to manage your sleep during Ramadan

During Ramadan, many Muslims around the world fast from sunrise to sunset. This can have an impact on your sleep patterns, as you may be eating and drinking at different times than usual, and staying up later for prayer and social gatherings.

Here are some tips to help manage your sleep during Ramadan:

1. **Maintain a regular sleep schedule:** Try to go to bed and wake up at the same time every day, even during Ramadan. This will help regulate your body's internal clock and ensure that you get enough rest.

2. **Take a nap:** If you feel tired during the day, take a short nap to help refresh your mind and body. However, be careful not to nap too close to iftar time, as this may make it harder for you to fall asleep at night.

3. **Avoid caffeine and sugar:** Both caffeine and sugar can disrupt your sleep patterns, so it's best to avoid them during Ramadan. Instead, drink plenty of water and eat healthy, nutritious foods that will help sustain your energy levels throughout the day.

4. **Create a relaxing bedtime routine:**
    Before going to bed, take some time to
    relax and unwind. This could include
    reading a book, taking a warm bath, or
    practicing some gentle yoga or
    stretching exercises.

5. **Make your bedroom comfortable:**
    Ensure that your bedroom is cool, quiet,
    and dark to promote restful sleep. Use
    blackout curtains or an eye mask to
    block out any light, and consider using a
    white noise machine or earplugs to
    block out any noise.

By following these tips, you can help ensure
that you get enough restful sleep during
Ramadan, which will help you stay energized
and focused throughout the day.

How Supplementation can help when fasting

Alongside your training, nutrition and lifestyle
changes, supplementation can be helpful to
plug any gaps.

- Magnesium can help calm the nervous
  system and promote restful sleep.

- Whey protein powder is fast and easily digestible and can help with hitting protein intake targets.

- With a very short eating window, digestive enzymes can help improve digestion.

- Chocotrients is a chocolate greens powder full of nutrients to support your immune system, and it's delicious!

Does fasting in Ramadan help lose weight?

Fasting during Ramadan may lead to weight loss for some people, but it is not a guaranteed method for losing weight.

During Ramadan, Muslims fast from sunrise to sunset, which typically lasts for about 12-16 hours depending on the location.

This means that they will consume all of their daily calories during a shorter period of time, which can create a calorie deficit and potentially lead to weight loss.

However, it is important to note that weight loss during Ramadan will depend on several factors, including the individual's diet, activity level, and overall health.

 It is also important to maintain a balanced and nutritious diet during the non-fasting hours to avoid overeating and consuming unhealthy foods, which can negate any potential weight loss.

Moreover, fasting during Ramadan is primarily a religious practice, and any potential weight loss should not be the sole reason for observing the fast.

It is important to consult with a healthcare provider or a registered dietitian if you have any concerns about your health or diet during Ramadan.

Is fermented foods good for you during fasting period

Fermented foods can be a beneficial addition to your diet during fasting periods, as they offer several potential health benefits.

Fermented foods are those that have been preserved through the process of lacto-fermentation, which involves the use of bacteria or yeast to break down sugars and produce lactic acid. Examples of fermented foods include yogurt, kefir, kimchi, sauerkraut, miso, and kombucha.

During fasting periods, fermented foods can provide a source of probiotics, which are beneficial bacteria that can help support digestion and boost the immune system. Additionally, fermented foods may help improve gut health and reduce inflammation in the body.

However, it is important to note that some fermented foods, such as kimchi and sauerkraut, may be high in sodium, which can lead to dehydration during fasting periods. It is important to consume these foods in moderation and drink plenty of water to stay hydrated.

Fermented foods can be a healthy addition to your diet during fasting periods, but it is important to consume them in moderation and to ensure that you are also getting enough hydration and nutrients from other sources.

Chapter 7

The Importance of Laylat Al-Qadr

what is Laylat Al-Qadr

Laylat Al-Qadr is a special night in the Islamic faith that occurs during the last ten days of the holy month of Ramadan. It is also known as the Night of Power or the Night of Destiny.

According to Islamic teachings, this night is considered to be the most significant night of the year, as it is believed to be the night when the first verses of the Quran were revealed to the Prophet Muhammad (peace be upon him).

Muslims believe that Laylat Al-Qadr is a night of great spiritual significance, and it is believed that acts of worship performed on this night are worth more than a thousand months of worship.

Therefore, many Muslims spend the night in prayer and supplication, seeking forgiveness, and asking for blessings and guidance from Allah (God).

The exact date of Laylat Al-Qadr is not known, but it is believed to fall on one of the odd-numbered nights during the last ten days of Ramadan, which are the 21st, 23rd, 25th, 27th, or 29th night of Ramadan.

Muslims are encouraged to seek out this special night by staying up late in prayer, reading the Quran, and making supplications to Allah.

How to observe Laylat Al Qadr

Observing Laylat Al-Qadr is an important aspect of Ramadan for Muslims. Here are some ways that Laylat Al-Qadr can be observed:

1. Offer night prayers (Taraweeh): Muslims should perform the night prayers (Taraweeh) during the last ten nights of Ramadan, especially on odd-numbered nights such as the 21st, 23rd, 25th, 27th, or 29th night.

    They can perform these prayers individually or in congregation in a mosque or at home.

2. Recite Quran: Muslims can recite and reflect on the Quran during Laylat Al-Qadr. The Quran is believed to have been revealed on this night, so reciting it and

reflecting on its meaning is considered a way to draw closer to Allah.

3. Make dua (supplication): Muslims can make dua during Laylat Al-Qadr, seeking forgiveness, guidance, and blessings from Allah.

4. Engage in Dhikr (remembrance of Allah): Muslims can engage in Dhikr, which involves remembering Allah through recitation of His names and praises.

5. Perform good deeds: Muslims are encouraged to perform good deeds during Laylat Al-Qadr, such as giving to charity, helping others, and being kind and compassionate towards others.

6. Stay awake: Muslims are encouraged to stay awake during the last ten nights of Ramadan, especially on odd-numbered nights, in order to seek out Laylat Al-Qadr. They can engage in worship, recitation of Quran, and reflection during this time.

Observing Laylat Al-Qadr is a way for Muslims to seek forgiveness, guidance, and blessings from Allah, and to increase their spirituality and draw closer to Him.

What Quran says about Laylat Al Qadr?

The Quran mentions Laylat Al-Qadr in Surah Al-Qadr, which is the 97th chapter of the Quran. Here is the translation of the first few verses of this chapter:

"In the name of Allah, the Most Gracious, the Most Merciful.

1. Indeed, We sent the Quran down during the Night of Decree.

2. And what can make you know what is the Night of Decree?

3. The Night of Decree is better than a thousand months.

4. The angels and the Spirit descend therein by permission of their Lord for every matter.

5. Peace it is until the emergence of dawn." (Quran 97:1-5)

These verses indicate the significance of Laylat Al-Qadr in the Islamic faith, and that it is a night of great importance and blessings.

Muslims are encouraged to seek out Laylat Al-Qadr during the last ten nights of Ramadan and to engage in acts of worship, reflection, and supplication on this special night.

Hadiths on Laylat Al Qadr

There are several Hadiths (narrations of the sayings and actions of Prophet Muhammad) about Laylat Al-Qadr. Here are a few:

1. Abu Hurairah (May Allah be pleased with him) reported that the Prophet (ﷺ) said: "Whoever established prayers on the night of Qadr out of sincere faith and hoping for a reward from Allah, then all his previous sins will be forgiven; and whoever fasts in the month of Ramadan out of sincere faith, and hoping for a reward from Allah, then all his previous sins will be forgiven." (Bukhari and Muslim)

2. Aisha (May Allah be pleased with her) reported that the Prophet (ﷺ) said: "Search for the Night of Qadr in the odd nights of the last ten days of Ramadan." (Bukhari and Muslim)

3. Ibn Umar (May Allah be pleased with
    them) reported that the Prophet (Peace
    be upon him) and said: "The person who
    spends the night of Qadr in prayer out of
    faith and seeking reward from Allah,
    then all his previous sins will be
    forgiven." (Ibn Majah)

These Hadiths emphasize the importance of
seeking Laylat Al-Qadr during the last ten
nights of Ramadan, and the rewards that come
with engaging in acts of worship and
supplication on this special night.

**Why is laylatul qadr consider better than a
thousand months?**

Laylatul Qadr is considered better than a
thousand months because it is the night in
which the first verses of the Quran were
revealed to the Prophet Muhammad (peace be
upon him).

The Quran describes it as a night of great
importance and significance, with many
blessings and rewards for those who engage in
worship and good deeds.

The significance of Laylatul Qadr is emphasized in the Quran, where it is described as better than a thousand months:

"The Night of Decree is better than a thousand months." (Quran 97:3)

This means that any act of worship or good deed performed on Laylatul Qadr is equivalent in reward to performing the same act for over 83 years.

This is a great opportunity for Muslims to earn immense rewards and seek forgiveness for their sins.

Additionally, Laylatul Qadr is a night of peace and blessings, where angels descend to earth and the blessings of Allah are showered upon those who engage in worship and good deeds.

It is a night of intense spiritual reflection and connection with Allah, and many Muslims spend the night in prayer and contemplation.

The significance of Laylatul Qadr is rooted in its connection to the revelation of the Quran and the immense blessings and rewards associated with it.

What is I`tikaf?

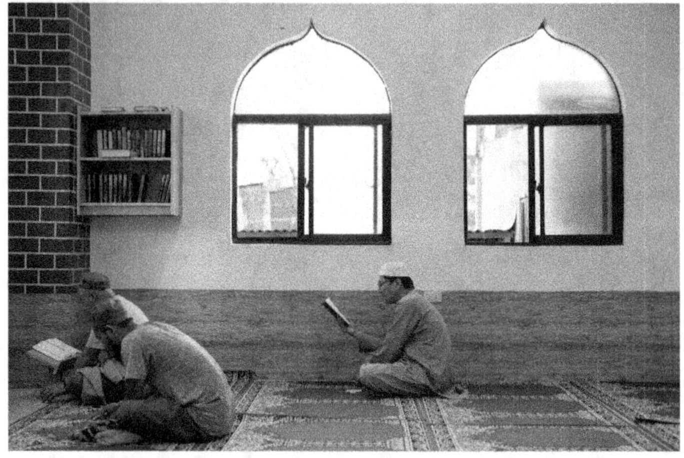

Itikaf is a voluntary spiritual retreat in Islam where a person secludes themselves in a mosque for a certain period of time, usually during the last ten days of Ramadan.

During this time, the person focuses solely on worship and spiritual activities, such as reading the Quran, engaging in prayer, and making supplications to Allah. Itikaf is considered a way to detach oneself from the distractions of the world and to deepen one's connection with Allah.

During I`tikaf, the person must stay within the confines of the mosque and may not leave except for a valid reason, such as using the restroom or performing ablution (ritual washing).

The person may also not engage in any worldly activities or conversations but rather must focus solely on spiritual pursuits.

I`tikaf is a voluntary act of worship and is not mandatory in Islam, but it is highly recommended, especially during the last ten days of Ramadan when Laylat Al-Qadr (the Night of Power) is believed to occur.

Voluntary Prayers (Salah)

Taraweeh prayer

Taraweeh prayer is a special type of prayer that is performed during the month of Ramadan, which is the ninth month of the Islamic lunar calendar.

 It is an additional prayer that is performed after the obligatory prayer of Isha and is usually performed in congregation in mosques.

Taraweeh prayer consists of 20 rak'ahs (units of prayer), and it is performed after the Isha prayer. The prayer is usually led by a skilled imam (prayer leader) who recites long portions of the Quran during each rak'ah.

The prayer is typically performed in a slow and deliberate manner, with the imam pausing to take breaks between each rak'ah.

The purpose of the Taraweeh prayer is to provide an opportunity for Muslims to spend more time in prayer and reflection during the month of Ramadan.

It is considered a highly meritorious act of worship, and many Muslims strive to attend Taraweeh prayer regularly during the month.

While Taraweeh prayer is not obligatory, it is highly recommended, and many Muslims choose to attend it in order to deepen their spiritual connection to God during the month of Ramadan.

In some communities, Taraweeh prayer is a social event, with families and friends gathering at the mosque to pray together and enjoy each other's company during the holy month.

Why do some people pray 8 rakats of Taraweeh?

The practice of performing eight rakats of Taraweeh prayer is based on the teachings and practices of some schools of Islamic thought.

While the majority of Muslims perform 20 rakats of Taraweeh prayer during Ramadan, some follow the opinion of certain scholars who consider eight rakats to be sufficient.

Those who choose to perform eight rakats of Taraweeh prayer often base their decision on a narration attributed to the Prophet Muhammad (peace be upon him) in which he stated that there are eight rakats of voluntary prayers to be performed in Ramadan after the obligatory Isha prayer.

While this narration is considered weak by some scholars of hadith, others consider it to be a valid basis for the practice of performing eight rakats of the Taraweeh prayer.

Additionally, some argue that performing eight rakats of Taraweeh prayer allows for more time for personal reflection and recitation of the Quran during Ramadan.

It is important to note that both the 20 rakats and eight rakats versions of the Taraweeh prayer are considered valid and acceptable by Islamic scholars and that the choice of which to perform is ultimately up to the individual.

The focus of the Taraweeh prayer is on increasing devotion to God and deepening one's spiritual connection during the holy month of Ramadan, regardless of the specific number of rakats performed.

How did 20 rakats of Taraweeh came to be?

The practice of performing 20 rakats of Taraweeh prayer during Ramadan is based on a longstanding tradition that dates back to the early Islamic period.

According to historical accounts, the practice of performing the Taraweeh prayer during Ramadan was established during the time of the second Caliph, Umar ibn al-Khattab (may Allah be pleased with him).

Umar noticed that Muslims were praying alone or in small groups during Ramadan, and he wanted to establish a way for Muslims to pray together in the congregation.

He, therefore, instructed the Muslims to gather in the mosque and to perform the Taraweeh prayer in the congregation.

Initially, the Taraweeh prayer was performed in a congregation without any specific number of rakats being set.

However, during the time of the third Caliph, Uthman ibn Affan (may Allah be pleased with him), the practice of performing 20 rakats of Taraweeh prayer was established.

Uthman is said to have based this number on the practice of the Prophet Muhammad (peace be upon him), who would pray 11 rakats of voluntary prayer during Ramadan.

Over time, the practice of performing 20 rakats of Taraweeh prayer became widespread among Muslims and was established as the standard practice for Taraweeh prayer during Ramadan.

Today, the vast majority of Muslims around the world perform 20 rakats of Taraweeh prayer during the holy month of Ramadan as a way to deepen their spiritual connection to God and increase their devotion during this special time of the year.

Salatul Tasbeeh

Salatul Tasbeeh is a voluntary prayer in Islam that involves the recitation of the Tasbeeh, a specific phrase that is repeated multiple times during the prayer.

The prayer is performed by Muslims in order to seek forgiveness for their sins and to increase their spiritual connection with Allah.

During the Salatul Tasbeeh, the worshipper recites the Tasbeeh phrase "Subhan Allahi wal hamdulillahi wa la ilaha illa Allahu wallahu akbar" (Glory be to Allah, praise be to Allah, there is no god but Allah, and Allah is the greatest) a total of 300 times, while performing a series of specific physical movements and postures.

It is important to note that the Salatul Tasbeeh is not a mandatory prayer in Islam, but rather a voluntary one that is highly recommended.

It is often performed during special occasions, such as the month of Ramadan, or on Fridays, as it is believed to be a means of gaining immense rewards and blessings from Allah.

Tahajjud prayers

Tahajjud is a voluntary prayer that is performed during the night after one has slept for some time. It is a highly recommended prayer in Islam, and it is considered one of the most virtuous acts of worship that a Muslim can perform.

The word "Tahajjud" comes from the Arabic root word "hajada," which means "to stay awake at night." The Tahajjud prayer is usually performed after the Isha prayer, and it can be performed in the early part of the night or the late part of the night, before the Fajr prayer.

The Tahajjud prayer is typically performed in sets of two units, called rak'ahs, and it can be performed alone or in a congregation.

Muslims can perform as many sets of Tahajjud as they wish, but it is recommended to perform at least two rak'ahs.

The Tahajjud prayer is a time for Muslims to reflect on their relationship with Allah, seek forgiveness for their sins, and ask for guidance and blessings. It is a time for spiritual reflection and a chance to draw closer to Allah.

Performing the Tahajjud prayer is a voluntary act of worship, and it is not mandatory like the five daily obligatory prayers.

However, it is highly recommended, and many Muslims make it a regular part of their worship routine.

Abu Huraira reported: The Messenger of Allah, peace and blessings be upon him, said, "Our Lord Almighty descends to the lowest heaven in the last third of every night, saying: Who is calling upon Me that I may answer him? Who is asking from Me that I may give him? Who is seeking My forgiveness that I may forgive him?" Source: Ṣaḥīḥ al-Bukhārī 1145, Ṣaḥīḥ Muslim 758

Salat al-Eid

Salat al-Eid, also known as Eid prayer, is a special prayer performed by Muslims on the morning of Eid ul-Fitr and Eid ul-Adha.

The prayer is typically performed in large congregations in mosques or open areas and consists of two Rak'ahs (units) of prayer, each with additional Takbirs (Allahu Akbar) and recitations.

Here are the general steps for performing Salat al-Eid:

1. **Intention:** As with any prayer in Islam, the worshipper begins by making the intention to perform the Eid prayer.

2. **Takbiratul Ihram:** The Eid prayer begins with the Takbiratul Ihram, which is the declaration of the intention to start the prayer. The worshipper raises their hands and says "Allahu Akbar" (Allah is the Greatest) to begin the prayer.

3. **First Rak'ah:** The first Rak'ah of the Eid prayer is performed in the same way as the first Rak'ah of any other prayer. The worshipper recites Surah Al-Fatiha followed by another Surah or verses from the Quran.

4. **Takbirs:** After the recitation, the worshipper raises their hands and says "Allahu Akbar" three times, followed by the Imam who will lead the prayer. This is known as the Takbiratul Eid.

5. **Khutbah:** After the first Rak'ah, the Imam delivers a Khutbah (sermon) which typically focuses on the importance of Eid and the significance of the occasion.

6. **Second Rak'ah:** After the Khutbah, the second Rak'ah of the Eid prayer is performed. The worshipper recites Surah Al-Fatiha followed by another Surah or verses from the Quran.

7. **Takbirs:** After the recitation, the worshipper raises their hands and says "Allahu Akbar" three times, followed by the Imam who will lead the prayer. This is known as the Takbiratul Eid.

8. **Tasleem**: After the completion of the second Rak'ah, the worshipper says the Tasleem (peace greeting) by turning their head to the right and saying "Assalamu alaikum wa rahmatullah" (Peace be upon you and the mercy of Allah), and then turning their head to the left and repeating the same words.

What are the physical benefits of salah?

Salah, or prayer, is an integral part of Islamic worship and is performed five times a day by Muslims around the world.

While the primary purpose of Salah is spiritual and religious, it also has numerous physical benefits for the human body. Some of these benefits include:

1. **Improving physical fitness:** Salah involves various physical movements, such as standing, bowing, and prostrating, which can help improve overall physical fitness and flexibility.

2. **Boosting circulation:** The physical movements involved in Salah can help increase blood flow and circulation throughout the body, which can help improve cardiovascular health and reduce the risk of heart disease.

3. **Strengthening muscles and joints:** The physical movements of Salah can help strengthen the muscles and joints in the body, particularly in the legs, arms, and back.

4. **Promoting relaxation:** Salah involves taking time out of the day to focus on prayer and spiritual reflection, which can help promote relaxation and reduce stress and anxiety.

5. **Enhancing mental clarity:** The practice of Salah can help clear the mind and enhance mental clarity, which can help improve cognitive function and focus.

6. **Improving posture:** The physical movements of Salah involve standing up straight and maintaining proper posture, which can help improve overall posture and reduce the risk of back pain and other related issues.

The physical benefits of Salah can contribute to a healthier, more balanced lifestyle, and can help individuals achieve greater overall physical and mental wellbeing.

What are the mental benefits of salah?

Salah, or prayer, is a form of worship that has numerous mental benefits for those who practice it regularly. Some of these benefits include:

1. **Stress relief:** Salah provides a sense of calm and peace that can help reduce stress and anxiety.

2. **Improved focus:** The practice of Salah requires concentration and focus, which can help improve mental clarity and enhance focus.

3. **Spiritual nourishment:** Salah is a form of spiritual nourishment that can help individuals feel a deeper sense of purpose and meaning in their lives.

4. **Greater self-awareness:** Salah involves introspection and self-reflection, which can help individuals become more self-aware and develop a greater understanding of themselves.

5. **Emotional balance:** The practice of Salah can help individuals regulate their emotions and develop a greater sense of emotional balance.

6. **Increased gratitude:** Salah involves expressing gratitude to Allah, which can help individuals develop a greater sense of appreciation for the blessings in their lives.

7. **Greater sense of community:** Salah is often performed in congregation, which can help individuals develop a greater sense of community and belonging.

The mental benefits of Salah can contribute to a healthier, more balanced lifestyle, and can help individuals achieve greater overall mental and emotional wellbeing.

What are the spiritual benefits of salah?

Salah, or prayer, is a fundamental act of worship in Islam that has numerous spiritual benefits. Some of these benefits include

1. **Strengthening the relationship with Allah:** Salah is a means of direct communication with Allah, and it can help individuals strengthen their relationship with Him.

2. **Purification of the soul:** Salah is a means of purifying the soul and seeking forgiveness for sins.

3. **Developing mindfulness:** Salah involves being fully present at the moment and focusing on one's relationship with Allah, which can help individuals develop mindfulness and spiritual awareness.

4. **Strengthening faith:** The practice of Salah can help individuals strengthen their faith in Allah and increase their devotion to Islam.

5. **Developing humility:** Salah involves humbling oneself before Allah, which can help individuals develop a greater sense of humility and gratitude.

6. **Developing patience and perseverance:** The regular practice of Salah requires discipline and commitment, which can help individuals develop patience and perseverance in other areas of their lives.

7. **Encouraging good deeds:** Salah is a means of encouraging good deeds and actions, and it can help individuals become more mindful of their actions and their impact on others.

The spiritual benefits of Salah can contribute to a deeper sense of purpose and meaning in life and can help individuals cultivate a greater sense of spirituality and devotion to Allah.

Chapter 8

Giving Charity Zakat and Fitra

Eid ul Fitr, also known as the Festival of Breaking the Fast, is an important Islamic holiday that marks the end of the holy month of Ramadan. It is celebrated on the first day of Shawwal, the tenth month of the Islamic calendar, following the sighting of the new moon.

During Ramadan, Muslims fast from dawn until sunset, abstaining from food, drink, and other physical needs. Eid ul Fitr is a time of celebration, as Muslims around the world come together to celebrate the end of this period of fasting and spiritual reflection.

On the morning of Eid ul Fitr, Muslims gather in mosques or open spaces for special prayers, known as Salat al-Eid. They dress in their finest clothes and offer thanks to Allah for the blessings and guidance received during the month of Ramadan.

Many Muslims also give charity to those in need, known as Zakat al-Fitr, before the Eid prayers.

Following the prayers, Muslims typically spend the day celebrating with family and friends, enjoying festive meals, and exchanging gifts.

Eid ul Fitr is a time of joy and celebration, marking the end of a period of sacrifice and devotion, and the beginning of a new month filled with blessings and opportunities for growth.

Giving charity (Zakat)

Giving charity (known as "zakat" in Islam) is an important part of Ramadan and is encouraged for those who are able to do so.

Muslims are required to give a portion of their wealth to those in need, typically 2.5% of their total savings and assets.

During Ramadan, many Muslims choose to increase their charitable giving as a way of purifying their souls and giving back to the community.

Giving charity while fasting in Ramadan is considered a particularly virtuous act, as it demonstrates a person's commitment to serving others despite their own hunger and thirst. It is believed that charitable acts are rewarded more generously during Ramadan and that giving charity can help bring a person closer to God and increase their spiritual growth.

There are many ways to give charity during Ramadan, including donating money to a charity or cause, volunteering at a local food bank or shelter, or helping a neighbor or friend in need.

Muslims are also encouraged to give "iftar" (the meal eaten after sunset to break the fast) to others, whether it be a friend, family member, or stranger in need.

Giving charity while fasting in Ramadan is an important way to show compassion and generosity towards others, and to strengthen one's faith and connection to the community.

Who are eligible for Zakat

Zakat is an obligatory form of charity in Islam, and it is given to those in need who meet certain criteria. According to Islamic teachings, there are eight categories of people who are eligible to receive Zakat:

1. **The poor:** Those who have little or no income, and are struggling to meet their basic needs.

2. **The needy:** Those who have some income, but it is not enough to cover their basic need.

3. **The destitute:** Those who have no source of income or support and are unable to meet their basic needs.

4. **Those employed to collect Zakat:** People who are employed by Islamic authorities to collect and distribute Zakat.

5. **Converts to Islam:** New Muslims who are in need of financial assistance.

6. **Those in debt:** People who are in debt and cannot pay it off, and need help to become debt-free.

7. **Those stranded while traveling:** Travelers who are stranded due to financial difficulties, and need assistance to continue their journey.

8. **Those fighting in the path of Allah:**
    Muslims who are fighting for a just
    cause, and need financial support for
    their cause.

Can Zakat be given to Non-Muslims?

Zakat is an obligation for Muslims to give to
those in need, who meet certain criteria as
mentioned in the above text.

 According to Islamic teachings, Zakat cannot
be given to non-Muslims, except in very
specific circumstances.

However, Muslims are allowed to give
voluntary charity, known as "sadaqah", to
non-Muslims as an act of kindness and
goodwill.

Sadaqah can be given to anyone, regardless of
their religion or background, and it is not
subject to the same rules and restrictions as
Zakat.

In fact, Islam encourages Muslims to be
generous and kind to all people, regardless of
their religion or ethnicity.

The Prophet Muhammad (peace be upon him) said, "Charity is prescribed for each descendant of Adam every day the sun rises.

To administer justice between two people is charity; to assist a man upon his mount, lifting him onto it or hoisting up his belongings onto it is charity; and to remove a troublesome object from the road is charity." (Bukhari, Muslim)

Therefore, while Zakat cannot be given to non-Muslims, Muslims are encouraged to give voluntary charity to all those in need, regardless of their faith.

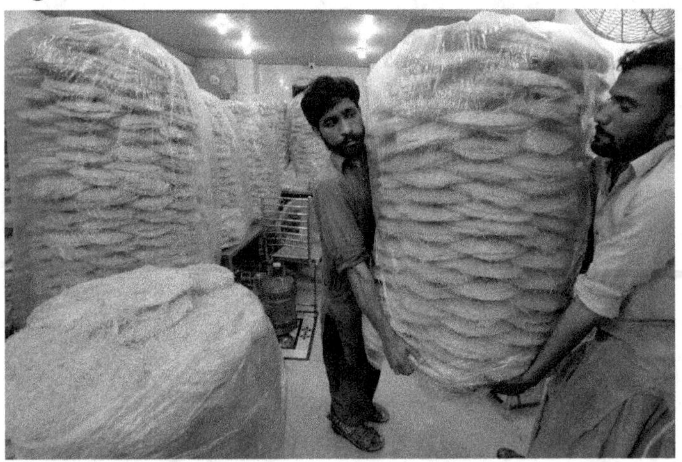

What is a fitra?

Fitra, also known as Zakat al-Fitr, is an obligatory charity given by Muslims at the end of the month of Ramadan, before the Eid al-Fitr prayer.

It is a means of purifying one's fast and a way to provide for the needs of the poor and needy in the community.

The purpose of Fitra is to ensure that all Muslims, regardless of their financial status, can celebrate Eid al-Fitr with dignity and happiness.

The amount of Fitra is usually based on the cost of one measure of food, such as wheat or barley, in the local area.

 It is recommended to give Fitra before the Eid prayer so that it reaches those in need before the start of the celebrations.

According to Islamic teachings, the payment of Fitra is obligatory on every Muslim who possesses food in excess of their needs and the needs of their dependents on the day of Eid al-Fitr.

The amount of Fitra is generally calculated as the price of one meal or food item, which can vary depending on the region and local customs.

Fitra is distributed to the poor and needy so that they can also enjoy the festivities of Eid al-Fitr.

The payment of Fitra is considered an act of worship and a way to seek Allah's pleasure and forgiveness for the shortcomings of the month of Ramadan.

Fitra is an important part of the celebration of Eid al-Fitr and a means of fulfilling the Islamic duty of helping those in need.

Who Should Pay al-Fitra?

The payment of Zakat al-Fitr is obligatory for every Muslim man, woman, adult, or the elderly, provided that they possess excess food or wealth that should not harm them financially.

If you are the head of your family. You should pay Zakat al-Fitr on behalf of each family member who is dependent on you..

When fitra should be paid?

Fitra, also known as Zakat al-Fitr, should be paid before the Eid al-Fitr prayer. The time frame for paying Fitra starts from the sunset of the last day of Ramadan until the time of the Eid prayer.

It is recommended to pay Fitra early enough so that the needy can benefit from it and enjoy the festivities of Eid al-Fitr.

However, it is permissible to pay Fitra in advance during Ramadan, or even a few days before the end of the month of Ramadan.

It is important to note that the obligation of Fitra falls on every Muslim who possesses food in excess of their needs and the needs of their dependents on the day of Eid al-Fitr.

The amount of Fitra is usually based on the cost of one measure of food, such as wheat or barley, in the local area. The amount can vary depending on the region and local customs.

Paying Fitra is an important aspect of the celebration of Eid al-Fitr, as it allows Muslims to fulfill their religious obligation of helping those in need and sharing their blessings with others.

Chapter 9

Favorite Ramadan food dishes from around the world:

1. **Fattoush Salad** - a Lebanese salad that includes fresh vegetables, crispy pita chips, and a tangy dressing

2. **Haleem** - a slow-cooked stew of lentils, wheat, and meat, popular in India, Pakistan, and the Middle East.

3. **Harira -** a soup made from tomatoes, lentils, and chickpeas, typically eaten to break the fast in Morocco.

4. **Kebabs** - various types of grilled or skewered meat, chicken, or vegetables that are popular in many Muslim countries.

5. **Biryani** - a flavorful rice dish that includes meat or vegetables and is popular in South Asia and the Middle East.

6. **Sambusa** - a savory fried pastry filled with meat or vegetables that is popular in East Africa and the Middle East.

7. **Foul medammes** - a traditional Egyptian dish made from fava beans, often served for breakfast during Ramadan.

8. **Katayef** - a sweet pastry filled with cream or nuts, typically eaten as a dessert during Ramadan in the Middle East and North Africa.

9. **Turkish Delight** - a type of sweet confectionery made with sugar, cornstarch, and flavorings that is popular throughout the Middle East.

These are just a few examples, and there are many more delicious and traditional Ramadan dishes enjoyed around the world.

Delicious recipes and meal plans for suhoor and iftar:

Here are some delicious recipes and meal plans for suhoor and iftar during Ramadan:

Suhoor meal ideas:

- Oatmeal with sliced bananas and honey
- Scrambled eggs with spinach and feta cheese, whole wheat toast
- Greek yogurt with granola and berries
- Avocado toast with smoked salmon
- Whole grain cereal with almond milk, fresh fruit
- Vegetable omelet with whole wheat pita bread

Iftar meal ideas:

- Lentil soup with whole grain bread
- Chicken kebabs with hummus and tabbouleh salad
- Grilled fish with roasted vegetables and quinoa
- Beef stir-fry with brown rice and steamed broccoli
- Baked sweet potato with black beans and salsa
- Chickpea curry with whole wheat naan bread

It's important to balance your meals with protein, complex carbohydrates, and healthy fats to keep you feeling full and energized throughout the day. Don't forget to also stay hydrated by drinking plenty of water and other fluids during non-fasting hours.

The Prophet Muhammad (peace be upon him) also emphasized the importance of moderation during Ramadan.

He encouraged Muslims to eat and drink in moderation during the evening meal (iftar) and to avoid overeating, as this can lead to health problems and distract from the spiritual benefits of fasting.

The Prophet Muhammad (peace be upon him) was a role model for Muslims in terms of his commitment to fasting and his emphasis on the spiritual benefits of this practice.

His example continues to inspire Muslims around the world to fast regularly and to seek closeness to God through acts of worship and devotion.

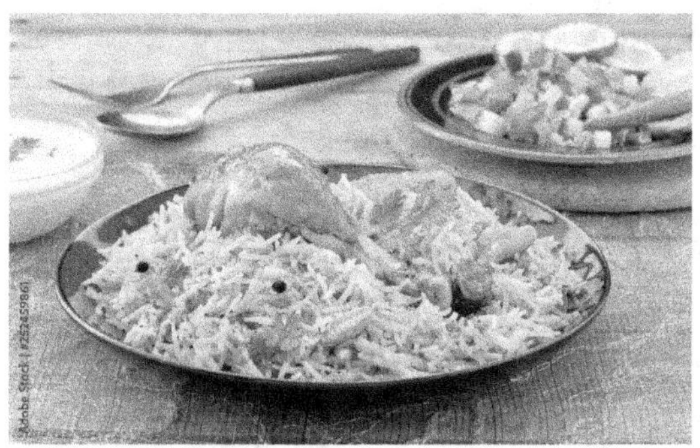

How to prepare pakora

Pakoras are a popular snack in South Asian cuisine that can be enjoyed as an appetizer or as a tea-time snack. Here's a simple recipe for making pakoras at home:

Ingredients:

- 1 cup besan (chickpea flour)
- 1/2 tsp baking powder
- 1/2 tsp red chili powder
- 1/2 tsp turmeric powder
- 1/2 tsp cumin seeds
- 1/2 tsp salt
- 1/2 cup water (or as needed)
- 1 medium-sized onion, finely sliced
- 2-3 green chilies, finely chopped (optional)

- Handful of fresh coriander leaves, chopped
- Oil for frying

Instructions:

1. In a mixing bowl, add the besan, baking powder, red chili powder, turmeric powder, cumin seeds, and salt. Mix everything together.

2. Gradually add water to the mixture to form a smooth batter. The batter should be thick enough to coat the vegetables.

3. Add the sliced onions, chopped green chilies, and chopped coriander leaves to the batter. Mix everything together.

4. Heat oil in a deep frying pan over medium heat.

5. Using a spoon, drop small portions of the pakora batter into the hot oil. Fry the pakoras for 2-3 minutes on each side or until they turn golden brown.

6. Remove the pakoras from the oil using a slotted spoon and place them on a paper towel to drain the excess oil.

7. Serve hot with mint chutney, tamarind chutney, or ketchup.

Enjoy your homemade pakoras as a delicious snack or appetizer!

How to prepare haleem

Haleem is a popular and delicious slow-cooked stew made from lentils, wheat, and meat. Here's a recipe on how to prepare it:

Ingredients:

- 1 cup boneless beef or lamb
- 1 cup of lentils
- 1 cup of wheat grains
- 1 onion, finely chopped
- 2 teaspoons ginger garlic paste
- 1 teaspoon turmeric powder
- 1 teaspoon red chili powder
- 1 teaspoon cumin powder
- 1 teaspoon coriander powder
- Salt to taste
- 1/4 cup oil
- 1 lemon, cut into wedges
- 2 tablespoons fresh coriander leaves, chopped

Instructions:

1. Soak the lentils and wheat grains separately for at least 6 hours or overnight.
2. In a large pot, add the meat, lentils, and wheat along with 6 cups of water. Cook on low heat until the meat and grains are tender and cooked through. This could take anywhere from 2 to 4 hours.

3. Once the meat and grains are cooked, use a hand blender or mash the mixture with a potato masher to form a smooth consistency.

4. In a separate pan, heat the oil and add the chopped onion. Fry the onion until it turns golden brown.

5. Add the ginger garlic paste and fry for 2 minutes.

6. Add the turmeric powder, red chili powder, cumin powder, coriander powder, and salt. Fry for 1-2 minutes.

7. Add the meat and lentil mixture to the pan with the fried spices and onions.

Mix well and cook for an additional 10-15 minutes, stirring frequently.

8. Garnish with fresh coriander leaves and lemon wedges before serving.

Haleem is typically served hot with naan bread or rice. Enjoy!

How to Prepare Harira

Harira is a traditional soup that is commonly eaten to break the fast during Ramadan in Morocco. It's a hearty and flavorful soup made with lentils, chickpeas, tomatoes, and a variety of spices. Here's a recipe on how to prepare it:

Ingredients:

- 1/2 cup dried chickpeas, soaked overnight
- 1/2 cup red lentils
- 1 onion, finely chopped
- 1 teaspoon ginger, grated
- 2 cloves garlic, minced
- 1/2 teaspoon turmeric powder
- 1/2 teaspoon cinnamon powder
- 1/2 teaspoon cumin powder
- 1/2 teaspoon paprika

- 1/2 teaspoon black pepper
- 2 tablespoons tomato paste
- 1 can (400g) diced tomatoes
- 6 cups water or vegetable broth
- Salt, to taste
- 1/4 cup fresh parsley, chopped
- 1/4 cup fresh cilantro, chopped
- 2 tablespoons lemon juice

Instructions:

1. In a large pot, add the soaked chickpeas and 6 cups of water. Bring to a boil, then reduce heat to low and simmer for 30 minutes.

2. Add the red lentils to the pot and continue to simmer for an additional 15 minutes.

3. In a separate pan, heat 2 tablespoons of oil and sauté the onion, ginger, and garlic until the onion is translucent.

4. Add the turmeric powder, cinnamon powder, cumin powder, paprika, and black pepper to the onion mixture. Stir for 1-2 minutes.

5. Add the tomato paste and diced tomatoes to the onion mixture and stir well.

6. Add the onion and tomato mixture to the pot with the chickpeas and lentils. Mix well and cook for an additional 10-15 minutes.

7. Add salt to taste and adjust the thickness of the soup by adding water or broth as needed.

8. Just before serving, add fresh parsley, cilantro, and lemon juice. Stir well and serve hot.

Harira is typically served with dates and bread for breaking the fast during Ramadan. Enjoy!

How to prepare meat kabob

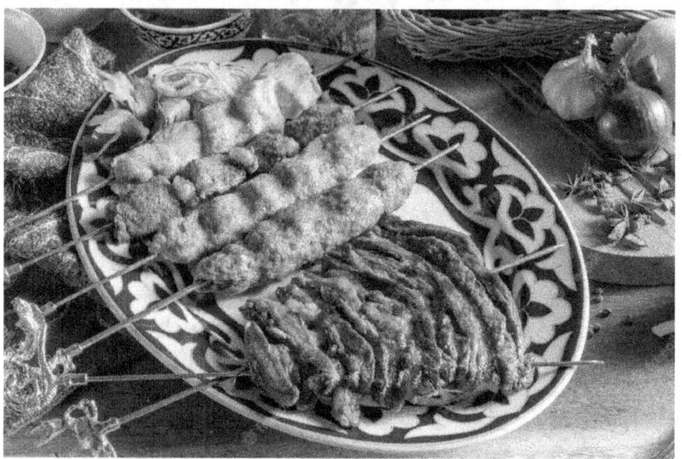

Meat kebab, also known as Shish Kebab, is a popular grilled meat dish made with marinated pieces of meat and vegetables. Here's a recipe on how to prepare it:

Ingredients:
- 1 lb. beef or lamb, cut into 1-inch cubes
- 1 onion, chopped
- 1/4 cup olive oil
- 2 tablespoons lemon juice
- 2 teaspoons garlic, minced
- 1 teaspoon salt
- 1/2 teaspoon black pepper
- 1/2 teaspoon paprika
- 1/2 teaspoon cumin

- Vegetables such as bell peppers, onions, and tomatoes (optional)

Instructions:

1. In a large bowl, combine the chopped onion, olive oil, lemon juice, minced garlic, salt, black pepper, paprika, and cumin.

2. Add the meat to the marinade and toss to coat. Cover the bowl with plastic wrap and refrigerate for at least 2 hours or overnight for best results.

3. If using vegetables, cut them into 1-inch pieces and thread them onto skewers alternating with the marinated meat cubes.

4. Preheat the grill to medium-high heat. If using wooden skewers, soak them in water for 30 minutes before grilling.

5. Grill the skewers for 8-10 minutes on each side, or until the meat is cooked to your desired level of doneness.

6. Remove the skewers from the grill and
    let them rest for a few minutes before
    serving.

You can serve the meat kebab hot off the grill
with rice, bread, or a salad on the side. Enjoy!

How to Prepare Foul Medammes

Foul Medammes is a popular Middle Eastern
dish made from cooked fava beans, usually
served for breakfast or brunch. Here's a recipe
on how to prepare it:

Ingredients:

- 1 can (15 oz) cooked fava beans
- 1/4 cup olive oil
- 1/4 cup lemon juice
- 2 garlic cloves, minced
- 1 teaspoon cumin
- Salt, to taste
- Parsley, chopped (optional)
- Tomatoes, chopped (optional)
- Onion, chopped (optional)
- Hard-boiled eggs, sliced (optional)

Instructions:

1. Drain and rinse the canned fava beans in cold water, then transfer them to a pot.

2. Add enough water to the pot to cover the fava beans, and bring the water to a boil.

3. Reduce the heat to low and simmer the fava beans for about 10-15 minutes, or until they are soft.

4. In a separate bowl, mix together the olive oil, lemon juice, minced garlic, cumin, and salt.

5. Drain the cooked fava beans and transfer them to a serving bowl.

6. Pour the olive oil mixture over the fava beans and mix well.

7. Add chopped parsley, tomatoes, onions, and hard-boiled eggs on top of the fava beans, if desired.

8. Serve the foul medammes warm with bread or pita on the side.

Foul medammes can also be garnished with a sprinkle of sumac or a drizzle of olive oil before serving. Enjoy!

How to prepare Katayef

Katayef is a popular Middle Eastern dessert typically served during Ramadan. It's a sweet pastry that is similar to a mini pancake or crepe, filled with either cheese, nuts or cream. Here's a recipe on how to prepare the dough for the Katayef:

Ingredients:

- 2 cups all-purpose flour
- 2 tablespoons semolina flour
- 1 tablespoon instant yeast
- 1 tablespoon sugar
- 1/4 teaspoon salt
- 2 cups warm water
- 1/2 teaspoon baking powder
- 1/2 teaspoon vanilla extract

Instructions:

1. In a large mixing bowl, whisk together
    the all-purpose flour, semolina flour,
    instant yeast, sugar, and salt.

2. Gradually add in the warm water while
    stirring until you get a smooth, thin
    batter.

3. Add in the baking powder and vanilla
    extract and mix well.

4. Cover the bowl with a clean cloth and let
    the batter rest for 30 minutes.

5. Heat a non-stick pan over medium heat.

6. Using a small ladle, pour about 2
    tablespoons of the batter onto the pan,
    forming a small round circle about 3
    inches in diameter.

7. Cook the Katayef on one side until the
    top is dry and bubbly, then remove it
    from the pan and place it on a plate.

8. Repeat the process until all the batter is
    used up.

To make the filling for the Katayef:

- For cheese filling: mix together 1 cup of unsalted white cheese, such as ricotta cheese, with 1 tablespoon of sugar and 1/2 teaspoon of orange blossom water.

- For nut filling: mix together 1 cup of finely chopped nuts, such as walnuts or pistachios, with 1 tablespoon of sugar and 1/2 teaspoon of cinnamon.

To assemble the Katayef:

1. Take one cooked Katayef pancake and place a spoonful of the filling in the center.

2. Fold the pancake in half and pinch the edges together to seal it.

3. Repeat the process until all the pancakes are filled.

4. You can serve the Katayef either warm or at room temperature.

Katayef can also be served drizzled with honey or syrup and sprinkled with chopped nuts or powdered sugar. Enjoy!

How to prepare fattoush salad

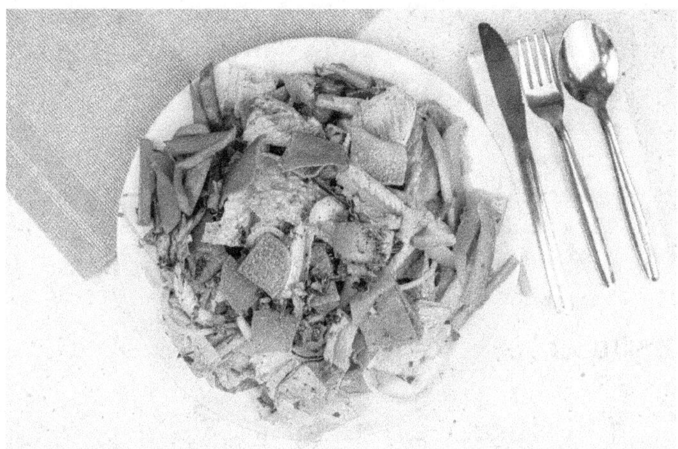

Fattoush is a traditional Middle Eastern salad that is popular during Ramadan. It's a refreshing and flavorful salad made with crispy pita bread, fresh vegetables, and a tangy dressing.

Here's a recipe on how to prepare Fattoush salad:

Ingredients:

- 2 pita breads, torn into bite-sized pieces
- 1 head of romaine lettuce, chopped
- 2 medium-sized cucumbers, diced
- 4 medium-sized tomatoes, diced
- 1 small red onion, sliced thinly
- 1/2 cup chopped fresh parsley

- 1/2 cup chopped fresh mint
- 1/2 cup chopped fresh cilantro
- 1/2 cup chopped radish
- 1/4 cup extra-virgin olive oil
- 1/4 cup lemon juice
- 1 garlic clove, minced
- 1 teaspoon sumac
- Salt and pepper, to taste

Instructions:

1. Preheat the oven to 350°F.

2. Spread the torn pita bread on a baking sheet and bake for 10-12 minutes until crispy.

3. In a large mixing bowl, combine the chopped lettuce, diced cucumbers, tomatoes, sliced red onion, chopped parsley, mint, cilantro, and radish.

4. Add the crispy pita bread to the salad and mix well.

5. In a separate mixing bowl, whisk together the extra-virgin olive oil, lemon juice, minced garlic, sumac, salt, and pepper.

6. Pour the dressing over the salad and toss well to combine.

7. Let the salad sit for 10-15 minutes before serving, allowing the pita bread to absorb the dressing.

You can also add other vegetables or herbs to the Fattoush salad such as chopped bell peppers, sliced olives, or diced avocado. Enjoy the fresh and tangy flavors of this delicious salad!

How to prepare Sambusa (Samosa)

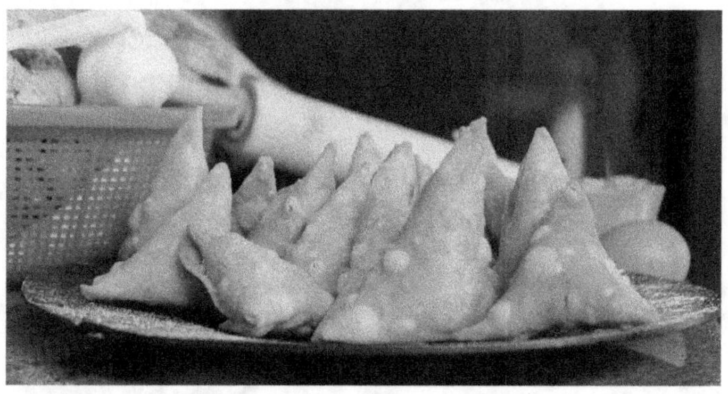

Sambusa, also known as samosa, is a popular appetizer in many countries, particularly in the Middle East, South Asia, and Africa.

It's a crispy pastry filled with savory ingredients such as spiced vegetables, meat, or cheese. Here's a recipe on how to prepare the dough and filling for vegetable Sambusa:

Ingredients for dough:

- 2 cups all-purpose flour
- 1/2 teaspoon salt
- 1/4 teaspoon turmeric powder
- 1/4 teaspoon baking powder
- 1/4 cup vegetable oil
- 1/2 cup warm water

Ingredients for filling:

- 2 cups chopped vegetables (such as carrots, potatoes, onions, and peas)
- 1 tablespoon vegetable oil
- 1 teaspoon cumin powder
- 1 teaspoon coriander powder
- 1/2 teaspoon turmeric powder
- Salt and pepper, to taste
- 2 tablespoons chopped fresh cilantro

Instructions:

1. In a large mixing bowl, whisk together the all-purpose flour, salt, turmeric powder, and baking powder.

2. Add the vegetable oil and mix well, until the mixture resembles coarse crumbs.

3. Gradually add in the warm water while stirring until you get a smooth, pliable dough.

4. Knead the dough for a few minutes until it's smooth and elastic.

5. Cover the dough with a clean cloth and let it rest for 30 minutes.

To make the filling:

1. Heat the vegetable oil in a pan over medium heat.

2. Add the chopped vegetables and sauté for 5-7 minutes until they are tender.

3. Add the cumin powder, coriander powder, turmeric powder, salt, and pepper, and mix well.

4. Add the chopped cilantro and mix well.

5. Remove the filling from heat and let it cool.

To assemble the Sambusa:

1. Take a small portion of the dough and roll it into a thin circle.

2. Cut the circle in half to make two semi-circles.

3. Take one semi-circle and fold it into a cone shape, sealing the edges by wetting them with water.

4. Fill the cone with a spoonful of the vegetable filling.

5. Wet the open edge of the cone with water and press it together to seal it.
6. Repeat the process until all the dough and filling are used up.

To cook the Sambusa:

1. Heat the vegetable oil in a deep frying pan over medium heat.

2. Fry the Sambusa in batches until they
    are golden brown and crispy.

3. Remove them from the oil and place
    them on paper towels to remove excess
    oil.

Serve the Sambusa hot with your favorite
chutney or sauce. Enjoy!

How to prepare Taco

Tacos are a popular Mexican dish that typically
consists of a corn or flour tortilla filled with
various ingredients such as seasoned meat,
beans, cheese, lettuce, and salsa.

Here's a recipe on how to prepare beef tacos:

Ingredients:

- 1 pound ground beef
- 1 tablespoon vegetable oil
- 1 small onion, diced
- 2 cloves garlic, minced
- 2 teaspoons chili powder
- 1 teaspoon ground cumin
- 1/2 teaspoon paprika

- Salt and pepper, to taste
- 8-10 soft corn or flour tortillas
- Toppings (shredded lettuce, diced tomatoes, shredded cheese, salsa, guacamole, sour cream, etc.)

Instructions:

1. In a large skillet, heat the vegetable oil over medium heat.

2. Add the diced onion and minced garlic and sauté for 2-3 minutes until the onion is soft and translucent.

3. Add the ground beef and cook, breaking it up with a wooden spoon, until browned and cooked through.

4. Add the chili powder, ground cumin, paprika, salt, and pepper, and mix well.
5. Reduce the heat to low and let the beef mixture simmer for 5-10 minutes until the flavors have blended.

To assemble the tacos:

1. Heat the tortillas in a dry skillet over medium heat for 1-2 minutes on each side until they are warm and pliable.

2. Spoon the beef mixture onto each tortilla, leaving room for toppings.

3. Add your desired toppings such as shredded lettuce, diced tomatoes, shredded cheese, salsa, guacamole, and sour cream.

Fold the tortilla over the filling and enjoy your delicious beef tacos! You can also use this recipe to make chicken, or vegetarian tacos by substituting the ground beef with your desired protein or vegetables.

How to prepare american apple pie

Apple pie is a classic American dessert that is typically made with a buttery crust and a sweet apple filling. Here's a recipe on how to prepare American apple pie:

Ingredients:

For the crust:

- 2 1/2 cups all-purpose flour
- 1 teaspoon salt
- 1 teaspoon sugar
- 1 cup unsalted butter, chilled and diced
- 1/4-1/2 cup ice water

For the filling:

- 6-7 cups thinly sliced, peeled apples (about 6-7 medium-sized apples)
- 2 tablespoons lemon juice
- 1/2 cup sugar
- 1/4 cup all-purpose flour
- 1 teaspoon ground cinnamon
- 1/4 teaspoon ground nutmeg
- 1/4 teaspoon salt
- 2 tablespoons unsalted butter, cut into small pieces

Instructions:

1. Preheat the oven to 375°F.

2. In a large mixing bowl, combine the flour, salt, and sugar.

3. Add the diced butter to the flour mixture and use a pastry cutter or your hands to

mix until the mixture resembles coarse crumbs.

4. Add 1/4 cup of ice water to the mixture and use a fork to combine. Add more ice water as needed until the dough comes together into a ball.

5. Divide the dough into two equal parts and shape into disks. Wrap each disk in plastic wrap and chill in the refrigerator for at least 30 minutes.

6. In a separate mixing bowl, combine the sliced apples, lemon juice, sugar, flour, cinnamon, nutmeg, and salt. Mix well.

7. Roll out one of the chilled dough disks on a lightly floured surface into a 12-inch circle. Transfer the dough to a 9-inch pie dish.

8. Add the apple mixture to the pie dish and distribute the butter pieces on top of the apples.

9. Roll out the second chilled dough disk into a 12-inch circle and place on top of

the apple mixture. Trim the edges and crimp the edges of the crust.

10. Use a sharp knife to cut several small slits in the top of the crust to allow steam to escape.

11. Bake the pie in the preheated oven for 45-50 minutes until the crust is golden brown and the filling is bubbly.

12. Let the pie cool for at least 30 minutes before serving. Serve warm with a scoop of vanilla ice cream.

Enjoy your delicious American apple pie!

How to prepare fish

Fish is a versatile and healthy protein that can be prepared in many ways, including grilling, baking, frying, and steaming. Here's a simple recipe on how to prepare baked fish:

Ingredients:

- 4 skinless fish fillets (such as cod, tilapia, or salmon)
- 2 tablespoons olive oil

- 1/2 teaspoon salt
- 1/4 teaspoon black pepper
- 1/4 teaspoon garlic powder
- 1/4 teaspoon paprika
- 1 lemon, sliced into wedges

Instructions:

1. Preheat the oven to 375°F.

2. Rinse the fish fillets with cold water and pat dry with a paper towel.

3. Brush both sides of the fish fillets with olive oil and place them in a baking dish.

4. In a small mixing bowl, combine the salt, black pepper, garlic powder, and paprika. Sprinkle the spice mixture over the fish fillets.

5. Place the lemon wedges on top of the fish fillets.

6. Bake the fish in the preheated oven for 15-20 minutes, depending on the thickness of the fillets, until the fish is cooked through and flakes easily with a fork.

7. Remove the fish from the oven and let it rest for a few minutes before serving.

You can serve the baked fish with your choice of sides such as steamed vegetables, rice, or a salad. You can also add additional seasonings and herbs such as dill, parsley, or thyme to customize the flavor to your liking.

How to fry a fish

Frying fish is a popular cooking method that results in a crispy and flavorful crust. Here's a recipe on how to fry fish:

Ingredients:

- 2-3 fish fillets (such as cod, tilapia, or catfish)
- 1/2 cup all-purpose flour
- 1/2 teaspoon salt
- 1/4 teaspoon black pepper
- 1/4 teaspoon garlic powder
- 1/4 teaspoon paprika
- 1/2 cup milk or buttermilk
- 1 egg
- 1 cup breadcrumbs or panko breadcrumbs
- Vegetable oil for frying

- Lemon wedges for serving

Instructions:

1. In a shallow dish, combine the flour, salt, black pepper, garlic powder, and paprika.

2. In another shallow dish, whisk together the milk or buttermilk and the egg.

3. Place the breadcrumbs or panko breadcrumbs in a third shallow dish.

4. Rinse the fish fillets with cold water and pat dry with a paper towel.

5. Dredge each fish fillet in the flour mixture, shaking off any excess.

6. Dip each floured fish fillet in the milk and egg mixture, making sure to coat both sides.

7. Coat the fish fillets with the breadcrumbs, pressing the breadcrumbs onto the fish to adhere.

8. Heat enough vegetable oil in a deep frying pan or skillet to cover the fish fillets.

9. When the oil is hot (about 350°F), carefully add the fish fillets to the pan. Fry the fish for 3-5 minutes on each side until golden brown and cooked through.

10. Remove the fish from the pan with a slotted spatula and place them on a paper towel-lined plate to drain any excess oil.

11. Serve the fried fish with lemon wedges and your choice of sides such as fries or coleslaw.

Note: Be careful when handling hot oil, and make sure to have a fire extinguisher on hand just in case.

How to steam fish

Steaming fish is a healthy and easy cooking method that results in a tender and flavorful dish. Here's a recipe on how to steam fish:

Ingredients:

- 2-3 fish fillets (such as salmon or sea bass)
- 1 lemon, sliced
- Salt and black pepper to taste
- Fresh herbs such as dill or parsley (optional)

Instructions:

1. Rinse the fish fillets with cold water and pat dry with a paper towel.

2. Season both sides of the fish fillets with salt and black pepper to taste.

3. Place a few slices of lemon on a heat-safe plate or steamer basket that will fit inside a pot or wok with a lid.

4. Place the fish fillets on top of the lemon slices.

5. If desired, sprinkle fresh herbs such as dill or parsley over the fish.

6. Add enough water to the pot or wok so that it reaches just below the steamer basket or plate.

7. Bring the water to a boil over high heat.

8. Once the water is boiling, carefully place the steamer basket or plate with the fish inside the pot or wok.

9. Cover the pot or wok with a lid and reduce the heat to low.

10. Steam the fish for 8-10 minutes or until the fish is cooked through and flakes easily with a fork.

11. Carefully remove the plate or steamer basket from the pot or wok and serve the fish hot with additional lemon wedges and your choice of sides such as steamed vegetables or rice.

If you don't have a steamer basket, you can improvise one by placing a heat-safe plate or dish inside a large pot with a few inches of water in the bottom.

Make sure the plate or dish is elevated above the water level so that the fish is not submerged.

How to Prepare Turkish Delight

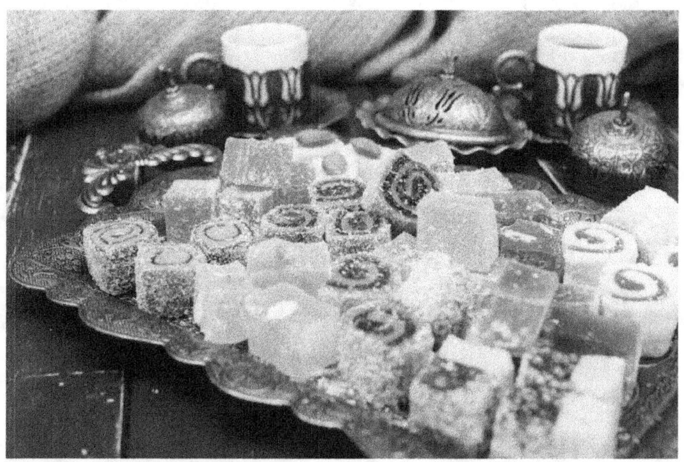

Turkish delight, also known as lokum, is a sweet confectionery made from starch and sugar syrup, often flavored with nuts, fruits, or spices. Here's a recipe on how to prepare traditional Turkish Delight:

Ingredients:

- 2 cups granulated sugar
- 2 cups water
- 1/4 cup lemon juice
- 1 cup cornstarch
- 1 teaspoon cream of tartar
- 1 teaspoon rose water
- Food coloring (optional)
- Powdered sugar, for coating

Instructions:

1. In a medium saucepan, combine the granulated sugar, water, and lemon juice. Cook over medium heat, stirring constantly, until the sugar has dissolved.

2. Bring the mixture to a boil and continue cooking, without stirring, until a candy thermometer inserted into the mixture reads 240°F (116°C).

3. In a separate bowl, whisk together the cornstarch and cream of tartar.

4. Gradually whisk the cornstarch mixture into the sugar syrup, stirring constantly to avoid lumps.

5. Continue cooking the mixture over low heat, stirring frequently, until it becomes thick and glossy, about 15-20 minutes.

6. Remove the pan from the heat and stir in the rose water and food coloring, if using.

7. Grease a shallow square or rectangular pan and pour the mixture into the pan.

8. Allow the Turkish Delight to cool to room temperature, then refrigerate for several hours or overnight until it is firm.

9. Cut the Turkish Delight into small squares using a sharp knife or a cookie cutter.

10. Coat each square in powdered sugar to prevent sticking.

11. Store the Turkish Delight in an airtight container at room temperature for up to 2 weeks.

You can customize the flavor and color of your Turkish Delight by using different extracts, nuts, fruits, or spices. Common variations include pistachio, almond, lemon, orange, cinnamon, and mint.

How to prepare Ramadan Pide

Ramadan pide is a traditional Turkish bread that is often eaten during the month of Ramadan. Here's a recipe on how to prepare it:

Ingredients:

- 4 cups all-purpose flour
- 2 teaspoons salt
- 2 tablespoons granulated sugar
- 1 tablespoon active dry yeast
- 1/4 cup warm water
- 1 1/4 cups warm milk
- 1/4 cup vegetable oil
- 1 egg, beaten
- Sesame seeds, for sprinkling

Instructions:

1. In a large mixing bowl, whisk together the flour, salt, and sugar.

2. In a separate small bowl, dissolve the yeast in the warm water and let it sit for 5-10 minutes until foamy.

3. Add the yeast mixture, warm milk, vegetable oil, and beaten egg to the flour mixture.

4. Mix the dough until it comes together into a smooth and elastic ball.

5. Cover the bowl with a damp towel and let the dough rise in a warm, draft-free

place for 1-2 hours, until it has doubled in size.

6. Preheat the oven to 400°F (200°C).

7. Punch down the dough and divide it into 8 equal pieces.

8. Roll each piece into a flat oval shape about 1/2 inch thick.

9. Use a sharp knife to make diagonal slashes across the top of each piece of dough.

10. Transfer the dough to a greased baking sheet.

11. Brush the tops of the dough with beaten egg and sprinkle sesame seeds over the top.

12. Bake the Ramadan pide for 15-20 minutes or until golden brown.

13. Serve the pide hot, sliced into wedges.

You can also add additional toppings to your Ramadan pide such as feta cheese, olives, or

herbs like oregano or thyme. Simply sprinkle
the toppings over the dough before baking.

Chapter 10

How is Eid al-Fitr celebrated?

Eid ul Fitr, also known as the Festival of Breaking the Fast, is an important Islamic holiday that marks the end of the holy month of Ramadan. It is celebrated on the first day of Shawwal, the tenth month of the Islamic calendar, following the sighting of the new moon.

Eid al-Fitr is an Islamic festival that marks the end of Ramadan, the month-long fasting period observed by Muslims around the world.

The celebration is a time of great joy and is characterized by special prayers, feasting, and exchanging of gifts among family and friends.

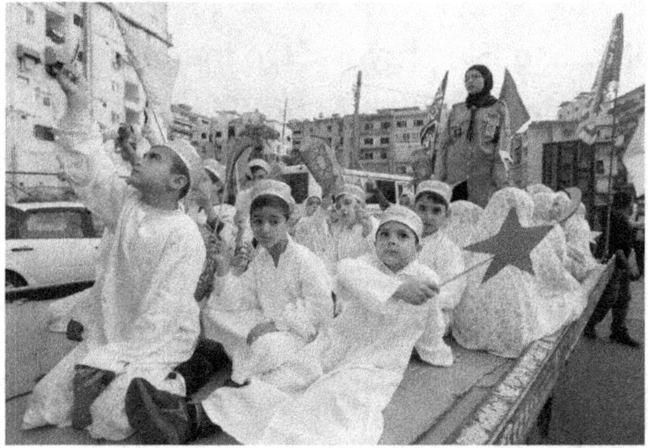

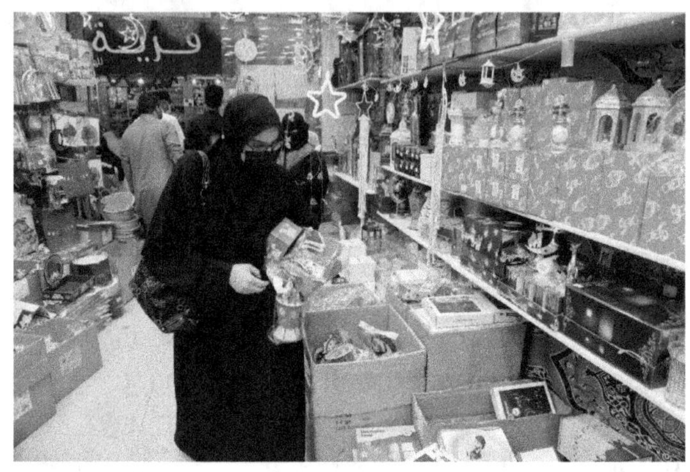

Here are some of the typical ways in which Eid al-Fitr is celebrated:

1. Preparing for the celebration: In the days leading up to Eid al-Fitr, Muslims clean their homes, buy new clothes, and shop for gifts and food items.

2. Attending Eid prayers: On the morning of Eid al-Fitr, Muslims gather in mosques or large open spaces to perform special Eid prayers. The prayers consist of two rak'ahs (units) and are led by an Imam.

3. Exchanging greetings: After the Eid prayers, Muslims greet each other with

the Arabic phrase "Eid Mubarak," which means "blessed Eid." They hug and shake hands as a sign of friendship and love.

4. Feasting: Eid al-Fitr is a time for feasting and sharing food with family and friends. Special dishes and sweets are prepared, and people invite each other over for meals.

5. Giving gifts: Muslims exchange gifts with each other, particularly with children, as a way of expressing love and gratitude.

6. Visiting relatives and friends: Eid al-Fitr is a time for visiting relatives and friends. Muslims often travel long distances to spend time with loved ones.

7. Giving to charity: Muslims are encouraged to give to charity during Eid al-Fitr. This can take the form of donating money, food, or other items to those in need.

Eid al-Fitr is a time of great celebration and joy for Muslims around the world. The religious Eid is the first and only day in the month of

Shawwal during which Muslims are not permitted to fast. The holiday celebrates the conclusion of the 29 or 30 days of dawn-to-sunset fasting during the entire month of Ramadan.

Eid al-Fitr is observed when the first new moon is sighted. This can lead to the festival being celebrated on different days in different parts of the world.

During Ramadan, Muslims fast from dawn until sunset, abstaining from food, drink, and other physical needs. Eid ul Fitr is a time of celebration, as Muslims around the world come together to celebrate the end of this period of fasting and spiritual reflection.

On the morning of Eid ul Fitr, Muslims gather in mosques or open spaces for special prayers, known as Salat al-Eid. They dress in their finest clothes and offer thanks to Allah for the blessings and guidance received during the month of Ramadan.

Many Muslims also give charity to those in need, known as Zakat al-Fitr, before the Eid prayers.

Following the prayers, Muslims typically spend the day celebrating with family and friends, enjoying festive meals, and exchanging gifts.

Eid ul Fitr is a time of joy and celebration, marking the end of a period of sacrifice and devotion, and the beginning of a new month filled with blessings and opportunities for growth.

What is the history of henna?

Henna is a natural dye made from the leaves of the henna plant, and has been used for thousands of years for cosmetic and medicinal purposes. The history of henna can be traced back to ancient cultures in the Middle East, North Africa, and South Asia.

The earliest recorded use of henna can be found in ancient Egyptian mummies, where the dye was used to decorate the hands and feet of both the living and the dead. It is also mentioned in ancient Indian texts, where it was used for various medicinal and cosmetic purposes.

Henna gained popularity as a cosmetic dye in the Middle East and North Africa, where it was used to decorate the hands and feet of brides and other women for special occasions. It was also used to create intricate designs and patterns on textiles, ceramics, and other decorative objects.

Over time, the use of henna spread to other parts of the world, including Europe and the Americas. In the 20th century, henna became a popular form of body art, particularly in the form of temporary tattoos.

In addition to its cosmetic uses, henna has also been used for its medicinal properties. It has been used to treat a variety of ailments, including headaches, skin disorders, and digestive issues.

Today, henna remains a popular cosmetic and medicinal product, particularly in the Middle East, North Africa, and South Asia.

It is still used for traditional bridal and celebratory decorations, as well as for temporary body art.

Henna is also used in hair dyes and other cosmetic products, and is often sought after for its natural and safe properties.

Who uses Henna

Henna is used by people of various cultures and religions around the world, but it is most commonly associated with cultures from the Middle East, North Africa, and South Asia.

In these regions, henna has been used for thousands of years for cosmetic, medicinal, and religious purposes.

In these regions, henna is often used to decorate the hands and feet of brides and other women for special occasions such as weddings, Eid festivals, and other celebrations.

It is also used for traditional body art, including temporary tattoos and intricate designs that are applied to the skin.

Henna is also used for medicinal purposes in these regions, and is believed to have anti-inflammatory, anti-fungal, and other therapeutic properties.

It is used to treat a variety of ailments, including headaches, skin disorders, and digestive issues.

In recent years, the use of henna has become more widespread, and it is now used by people from various cultures and backgrounds around the world.

It is particularly popular as a form of temporary body art and is often used as an alternative to permanent tattoos.

Henna is used by people from a wide range of cultures and backgrounds, and has a long and rich history of use for both cosmetic and medicinal purposes.

What is henna used for

Henna is a natural dye that has been used for thousands of years for various purposes. Here are some of the most common uses of henna:

1. **Cosmetic purposes:** Henna is perhaps best known for its use as a cosmetic dye. It is often used to decorate the hands and feet of brides and other women for special occasions such as weddings, Eid festivals, and other celebrations. Henna is also used to create intricate designs and patterns on textiles, ceramics, and other decorative objects.

2. **Body art:** Henna is a popular form of temporary body art, particularly in the form of temporary tattoos. These tattoos are often used for festivals, parties, or other special occasions, and can last for up to several weeks.

3. **Medicinal purposes:** Henna is believed to have a number of medicinal properties, and has been used for centuries to treat a variety of ailments. It is used to treat headaches, fever, skin disorders, and digestive issues, among other things.

4. **Hair care:** Henna is used in hair dyes and other hair care products. When applied to the hair, it can help to strengthen and condition the hair, and can also add a reddish or brownish tint.

5. **Spiritual and cultural practices:** Henna is often used in spiritual and cultural practices, particularly in the Middle East, North Africa, and South Asia. It is often used to mark special occasions such as weddings, religious festivals, and other celebrations.

Henna has a wide range of uses, from cosmetic to medicinal to cultural and spiritual. Its versatility and natural properties have made it a popular choice for people all over the world.

What are the benefits of henna?

Henna has a number of potential benefits, some of which have been supported by scientific research. Here are some of the potential benefits of henna:

1. **Natural hair dye:** Henna is a natural hair dye that is free of harsh chemicals and is often used to color hair. It can add a reddish or brownish tint to the hair and can also help to strengthen and condition the hair.

2. **Antimicrobial properties:** Henna has been found to have antimicrobial properties and may be effective against a range of bacteria, fungi, and viruses. This makes it a potential treatment for skin infections and other conditions caused by microorganisms.

3. **Anti-inflammatory properties:** Henna has been found to have anti-inflammatory properties and may be

effective in reducing inflammation and pain. This makes it a potential treatment for a range of conditions, including arthritis, headaches, and other inflammatory conditions.

4. **Skin and hair conditioning:** Henna can help to condition the skin and hair, leaving them feeling soft and moisturized. It can also help to improve the texture and appearance of the skin and hair.

5. **Cultural significance:** Henna has significant cultural and spiritual significance in many cultures around the world. Its use can help to promote cultural identity and traditions, and can also be a source of community and connection.

Henna has a range of potential benefits, both for cosmetic and medicinal purposes. While further research is needed to fully understand its effects, many people have found it to be a valuable addition to their beauty and wellness routines.

What are the side effects of henna?

While henna is generally considered safe, there are some potential side effects to be aware of. Here are some of the most common side effects of henna:

1. **Allergic reactions:** Some people may have an allergic reaction to henna, which can cause symptoms such as itching, swelling, and redness. In rare cases, henna can cause anaphylaxis, a severe allergic reaction that can be life-threatening.

2. **Skin irritation:** Henna can sometimes cause skin irritation, particularly if it is left on the skin for too long or if the skin is sensitive. Symptoms can include redness, itching, and burning.

3. **Staining of clothing and furniture:** Henna can stain clothing, furniture, and other surfaces. It is important to be careful when using henna and to protect your clothing and surroundings.

4. **Hair damage:** While henna is often used to strengthen and condition the hair, it can also cause damage if used

too frequently or left on the hair for too long. It is important to follow the instructions carefully and not to overuse henna.

5. **Chemical contamination:** Some henna products may be contaminated with harmful chemicals such as para-phenylenediamine (PPD), which can cause allergic reactions and other health problems.

It is important to be aware of these potential side effects and to use henna safely and responsibly. If you experience any adverse reactions, it is important to seek medical attention right away.

How to apply henna to hands

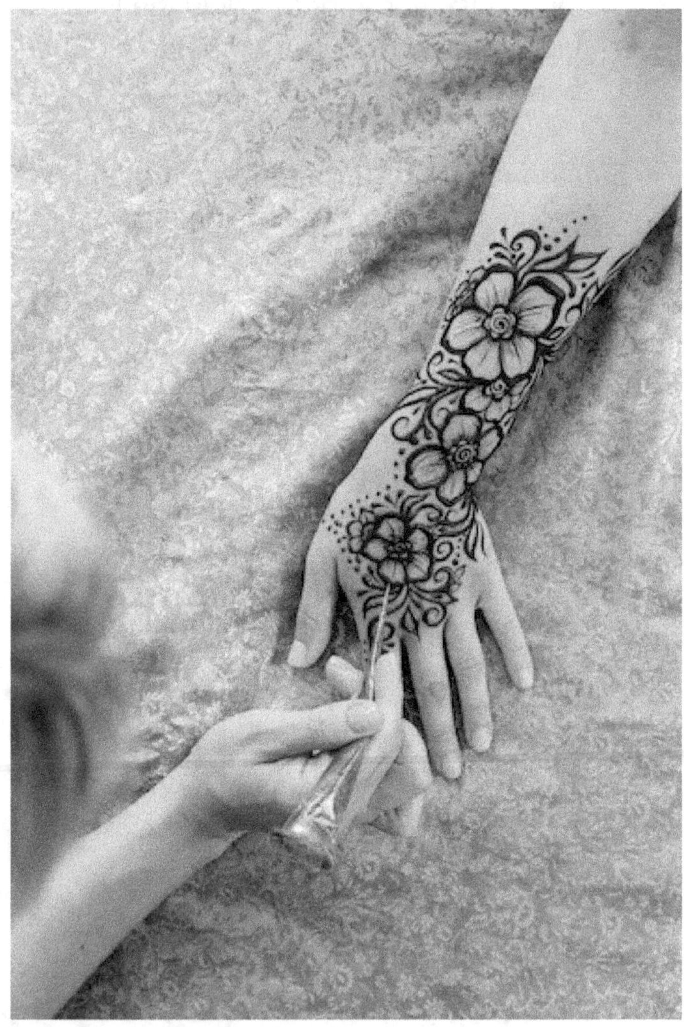

Applying henna to hands is a traditional art form and requires some practice to perfect.

Here are some general steps you can follow to apply henna to your hands:

1. **Prepare the henna paste:** Mix henna powder with lemon juice or water to create a paste that is smooth and easy to apply. Let the paste sit for a few hours to allow the dye to release.

2. **Clean and dry your hands:** Wash your hands thoroughly with soap and water to remove any dirt or oils. Dry your hands completely with a towel.

3. **Apply the henna paste:** Use a small plastic cone or a henna applicator bottle to apply the henna paste to your hands in the design of your choice. Start from the center of the palm and work your way outwards. Be careful not to apply too much pressure, as this can cause the paste to break or smudge.

4. **Allow the henna to dry:** Let the henna paste dry completely on your hands. This can take anywhere from a few hours to overnight, depending on the temperature and humidity.

5. **Remove the henna paste:** Once the henna paste is dry, gently scrape it off with a butter knife or your fingernails. Do not wash your hands with water for at least 12 hours, as this can affect the color and longevity of the henna.
6. **Seal the design:** To help the henna color last longer, you can apply a mixture of lemon juice and sugar to the design. This will help to seal the henna and make it more vibrant.

Remember that applying henna to hands is an art form, and it can take some practice to get the hang of it.

Be patient and take your time, and enjoy the beautiful designs you can create with henna.

How to apply henna to hair

Here are the general steps to apply henna to hair:

1. **Choose the right henna:** Make sure you choose a high-quality henna powder that is pure and free of additives or chemicals.

The color of the henna will depend on the quality and freshness of the powder.

2. **Prepare the henna paste:** Mix the henna powder with enough water to create a paste that is thick and smooth. Some people prefer to mix henna with lemon juice or tea to help release the dye.

3. **Section your hair:** Divide your hair into sections using clips or hair ties. This will make it easier to apply the henna evenly and thoroughly.

4. **Apply the henna paste:** Starting at the roots, apply the henna paste to your hair using a brush or your hands. Work your way through each section of your hair, making sure to coat the hair evenly with the henna.

5. **Cover your hair:** Once your hair is fully coated with henna, cover your hair with a shower cap or plastic wrap to help trap in heat and prevent the henna from drying out.

6. **Wait for the henna to set:** Leave the henna on your hair for at least 2-3 hours, or longer if you want a more intense color. You can also sit in the sun or use a hair dryer to help speed up the process.

7. **Rinse out the henna:** Once the henna has set, rinse your hair thoroughly with warm water. Do not use shampoo or conditioner, as this can strip the color from your hair. Rinse your hair until the water runs clear.

8. **Style your hair:** Once your hair is rinsed, you can style it as usual. Your hair may feel a bit dry or stiff at first, but this will improve with time.

Note that henna can be a bit messy to work with, so be sure to protect your clothing and surroundings. Also, henna can stain certain surfaces, so be careful when applying and rinsing out the henna.

How long is the effect of henna

The effect of henna on skin and hair can last for varying lengths of time depending on a few factors such as the quality of the henna, the strength of the mixture, and the location on the body.

When used as a temporary tattoo on skin, the color typically lasts for about one to two weeks before gradually fading away as the skin naturally exfoliates. The color may last longer on certain areas of the body that are less exposed to water and friction, such as the hands and feet.

When used on hair, the color can last for several weeks to a few months, depending on factors such as the initial color of the hair, the quality of the henna, and how well the henna is cared for after application.

Over time, the color will gradually fade away as the hair grows and is washed. The natural red-orange color that henna imparts on hair is known to be very long-lasting, and may even become more vibrant with multiple applications.

Chapter 11

What other days Muslims fast?

In addition to the obligatory fast of Ramadan, Muslims observe voluntary fasts on other days throughout the year. Here are some of the voluntary fasts observed by Muslims:

1. **The fast of Ashura:** This is the 10th day of the month of Muharram, the first month of the Islamic calendar. It commemorates the day when Allah saved the Prophet Moses and the Israelites from Pharaoh. Some Muslims fast on this day as a way to show gratitude and gain Allah's forgiveness.

    The fast of Arafat: This is the 9th day of the month of Dhul-Hijjah, the month of the Hajj pilgrimage. Muslims who are not performing the Hajj fast on this day as it is believed to expiate sins of the previous and coming year.

2. **The six days of Shawwal:** These are the six days following Eid al-Fitr, which is the celebration that marks the end of Ramadan. It is recommended for Muslims to fast for these six days as it is

believed to be equivalent to fasting for the entire year.

3. **Mondays and Thursdays:** It is a Sunnah to fast on these days as the Prophet Muhammad used to fast on these days regularly. It is also believed to have health benefits.

4. **The White Days:** These are the 13th, 14th, and 15th of each Islamic month, which correspond to the days of the full moon. Muslims who fast on these days believe that it is a way to gain Allah's blessings and forgiveness.

It's important to note that voluntary fasts are not obligatory, but rather a way for Muslims to increase their spiritual connection with Allah and gain blessings and rewards.

The fast of Ashura
The fast of Ashura is an important observance in the Islamic faith that falls on the 10th day of Muharram, the first month of the Islamic calendar. It is a voluntary fast that is highly recommended, but not obligatory.

The fast of Ashura has both historical and religious significance for Muslims. It is believed that on this day, Allah (God) saved Prophet Moses (Musa) and the Children of Israel from the Pharaoh of Egypt. It is also the day when Prophet Muhammad (PBUH) fasted to commemorate this event and encouraged his followers to do the same.

For Sunni Muslims, it is also a day to remember the martyrdom of the Prophet Muhammad's grandson, Imam Hussain (RA), and his family members at the Battle of Karbala in 680 CE. Shi'a Muslims mourn this event with public processions and gatherings.

The fast of Ashura is observed by abstaining from food and drink from dawn until sunset. Some Muslims also observe additional voluntary fasts on the 9th and 11th days of Muharram to distinguish their fast from the Jews who only fasted on the 10th day. It is also a day of charity, forgiveness, and doing good deeds.

The fast of Ashura is an important spiritual observance for Muslims and is a time to remember and reflect on important events in Islamic history.

The fast of Arafat is an Islamic observance that falls on the 9th day of the Islamic month of Dhu al-Hijjah, which is the month of the annual Hajj pilgrimage to Mecca. It is an important and highly recommended day of fasting for Muslims who are not performing the Hajj.

The fast of Arafat is closely associated with the Hajj, as it is the day on which the pilgrims gather on the plain of Arafat, located about 20 kilometers southeast of Mecca. It is considered the most important day of the Hajj, and pilgrims spend the entire day in prayer and supplication, seeking forgiveness and mercy from Allah (God).

For Muslims who are not performing the Hajj, fasting on the day of Arafat is believed to be a way to gain blessings and forgiveness from Allah. It is said that fasting on this day expiates the sins of the previous year and the coming year, and brings great rewards.

The fast of Arafat is observed by abstaining from food, drink, and sexual activity from dawn until sunset. It is also a day of prayer, charity, and doing good deeds. Muslims are encouraged to spend the day in prayer and supplication, seeking Allah's mercy and forgiveness.

The fast of Arafat is an important and highly recommended day of fasting for Muslims, whether they are performing the Hajj or not. It is a day of prayer, reflection, and seeking forgiveness from Allah, and is believed to bring great rewards and blessings.

The six days of Shawwal

The six days of Shawwal are a voluntary fasting period observed by Muslims after the month of Ramadan, which is the ninth month of the Islamic calendar. It is highly recommended but not obligatory to fast during these six days.

Muslims believe that fasting during the month of Ramadan is an obligation for all adult and healthy Muslims who are not traveling, but they can fast these six days of Shawwal to gain additional blessings and rewards from Allah (God).

The six days of Shawwal begin on the first day of Shawwal, which is the month that follows Ramadan. Muslims are encouraged to fast these six days consecutively, but it is also permissible to fast them separately throughout the month.

Fasting during these six days is considered to be equivalent to fasting for the entire year, as it is believed that Allah will reward the fasting person with a great reward for each day of fasting.

This is based on a hadith (a saying of Prophet Muhammad), where he said, "Whoever fasts Ramadan and follows it with six days of Shawwal, it will be as if he fasted for a lifetime."

The six days of Shawwal are also seen as a way to maintain the spiritual benefits gained during Ramadan and to continue the practice of fasting as a means of drawing closer to Allah.

Muslims are encouraged to use this time to reflect on their faith, strengthen their relationship with Allah, and engage in good deeds.

The six days of Shawwal are a voluntary fasting period that Muslims observe after Ramadan to gain additional blessings and rewards from Allah. Fasting during these days is highly recommended but not obligatory and is believed to be equivalent to fasting for the entire year.

It is also seen as a way to maintain the spiritual benefits gained during Ramadan and to continue the practice of fasting as a means of drawing closer to Allah.

Benefits of fasting in Shawwal

Fasting in the month of Shawwal, which comes immediately after Ramadan, has several benefits. Here are some of the benefits of fasting in Shawwal:

1. **Increases reward:** Fasting six days in Shawwal after the month of Ramadan brings immense reward. As per the authentic hadith mentioned earlier, fasting in Shawwal is equivalent to fasting for the whole year.

2. **Maintains the habit of fasting:** Fasting in Shawwal helps to maintain the habit of fasting, which is developed during Ramadan. It is an excellent way to continue the spiritual journey and stay connected to Allah.

3. **Detoxifies the body:** Fasting in Shawwal can help detoxify the body as it gives the digestive system a much-needed break. It also helps in reducing inflammation and can have a positive effect on overall health.

4. **Helps in weight loss:** Fasting in Shawwal can aid in weight loss, especially if done along with healthy eating and an active lifestyle.

5. **Boosts self-discipline and willpower:** Fasting requires self-discipline and willpower, which can be further strengthened by observing optional fasts in Shawwal.

The important benefit of fasting six days of Shawwal is that it makes up for any shortfall in a person's obligatory Ramadan fasts because no one is free of shortcomings or sins that have a negative effect on his fasting.

On the Day of Resurrection, some of his nafil deeds will be taken to make up for the shortcomings in his obligatory deeds.

Fasting in Shawwal has several benefits, including increased rewards maintaining the habit of fasting, detoxifying the body, aiding in weight loss, and boosting self-discipline and willpower.

Muslims should strive to observe these optional fasts to reap the benefits and continue their spiritual journey even after Ramadan.

What is the authentic hadith about Shawwal fasting?

The hadith about fasting in the month of Shawwal is reported by Abu Ayyub al-Ansari (may Allah be pleased with him) who said that the Prophet Muhammad (peace be upon him) said:

"Whoever fasts during the month of Ramadan and then follows it with six days of Shawwal will be rewarded as if he had fasted the entire year." (Sahih Muslim)

This hadith is considered authentic by scholars of hadith and is widely accepted as a basis for the recommendation to fast six days in the month of Shawwal.

It is important to note that this hadith does not make the six days of fasting in Shawwal obligatory, but rather voluntary, and the reward mentioned in the hadith is considered an encouragement for Muslims to fast these optional days.

Six Days of Shawwal or Missed Fasts: What Takes Priority?

According to Islamic teachings, it is recommended to observe six days of fasting in the month of Shawwal after the month of Ramadan.

However, if a Muslim has missed obligatory fasts during Ramadan, it is important to make up for those missed fasts before observing the optional fasts of Shawwal.

The priority should be given to making up for missed Ramadan fasts since they are obligatory while fasting in Shawwal is voluntary.

Once the missed Ramadan fasts have been made up, a Muslim can then observe the optional fasts of Shawwal.

It is important to note that a Muslim should not delay making up for missed Ramadan fasts until the following Ramadan.

It is recommended to make up for missed Ramadan fasts as soon as possible, and if a Muslim is unable to make up for missed fasts before the next Ramadan, they should give Fidya or Kaffara instead.

Making up for missed Ramadan fasts takes priority over observing the optional fasts of Shawwal.

Muslims should make up for missed Ramadan fasts as soon as possible and then observe the optional fasts of Shawwal.

Mondays and Thursdays

Mondays and Thursdays are considered auspicious days in Islamic tradition, and it is recommended for Muslims to fast on these days as a voluntary act of worship.

Prophet Muhammad (PBUH) used to fast on Mondays and Thursdays, and he recommended it to his followers. Fasting on these days is believed to have numerous spiritual benefits, including increased piety, strengthening of one's faith, and purification of the soul.

Fasting on Mondays and Thursdays is also seen as a way to follow the Sunnah (the traditions and practices of the Prophet Muhammad), and it is considered a good deed that brings reward from Allah (God).

It is important to note that fasting on Mondays and Thursdays is not obligatory, but it is a highly recommended act of worship. Muslims are free to choose which days to fast and can adjust their fasting schedule based on their personal circumstances.

In addition to fasting, Muslims are encouraged to engage in other acts of worship and good deeds on Mondays and Thursdays, such as reciting Quran, performing optional prayers, giving charity, and helping those in need.

In summary, fasting on Mondays and Thursdays is a voluntary act of worship that is highly recommended in Islamic tradition. It is believed to have numerous spiritual benefits and is seen as a way to follow the Sunnah of the Prophet Muhammad.

Muslims are free to choose which days to fast and are encouraged to engage in other acts of worship and good deeds on these days. It is mentioned in the hadith that on Monday the deeds are presented to Allah.

The White Days fasting
The White Days fasting refers to the voluntary fasting of the 13th, 14th, and 15th days of the Islamic lunar calendar, which correspond to the days when the moon is at its brightest and fullest.

These days are referred to as "Ayyam al-Bid" in Arabic, which means "the white days," and are believed to have significant spiritual significance in Islamic tradition.

Fasting on these days is considered to be a Sunnah (a practice of Prophet Muhammad) and is believed to bring numerous blessings and rewards.

Muslims are encouraged to fast on the 13th, 14th, and 15th days of each lunar month, and it is believed that fasting on these days is equivalent to fasting for a whole month.

This is based on a Hadith (a saying of Prophet Muhammad), in which he said, "Fasting three days of each month is equal to fasting for the whole year."

Fasting during the White Days is also believed to purify the soul, increase piety, and strengthen one's relationship with Allah (God).

It is also seen as a way to follow the Sunnah of Prophet Muhammad and to gain additional blessings and rewards from Allah.

It is important to note that fasting during the White Days is a voluntary act of worship and not an obligation in Islam.

Muslims are free to choose whether or not to fast on these days and can adjust their fasting schedule based on their personal circumstances.

In summary, the White Days fasting refers to the voluntary fasting of the 13th, 14th, and 15th days of the Islamic lunar calendar. Fasting on these days is considered a Sunnah and is believed to bring numerous blessings and rewards.

It is also seen as a way to purify the soul, increase piety, and strengthen one's relationship with Allah. However, fasting on the White Days is a voluntary act of worship and not an obligation in Islam.

What different types of fasting are there?

There are several different types of fasting, each with its own unique characteristics and potential benefits. Here are some of the most common types of fasting:

1. **Intermittent fasting:** This involves alternating periods of fasting and eating. The most common approach is to fast for 16-20 hours and eat during a 4-8 hour window. This can be done daily or a few times per week.

2. **Water fasting:** As mentioned earlier, this involves abstaining from all food and drinks except water for a specific period of time.

   Water fasting is an extreme form of fasting where a person abstains from all food and drinks, except for water, for a specific period of time. Water fasting is usually done for health or spiritual reasons, but it can also be done as a form of weight loss.

During water fasting, the body uses stored fat for energy instead of glucose from food. The process of using stored fat for energy is called ketosis, which can lead to rapid weight loss.

Water fasting can also lead to other potential health benefits, such as improved insulin sensitivity, reduced inflammation, and improved immune function.

However, water fasting is a highly restrictive and potentially dangerous practice that should only be done under medical supervision.

Water fasting can lead to dehydration, electrolyte imbalances, dizziness, fainting, and other health complications, especially if done for an extended period of time.

Water fasting is not suitable for everyone, especially individuals with certain medical conditions, such as diabetes, liver or kidney disease, and eating disorders.

It's important to consult a healthcare professional before attempting water fasting and to ensure that adequate hydration and electrolyte balance are maintained during the fasting period.

3. **Time-restricted eating:** This is similar to intermittent fasting, but the eating window is usually shorter, typically between 6-10 hours per day.

4. **Partial fasting:** This involves restricting certain types of food or nutrients, such as carbohydrates, protein, or fat, while still consuming other foods.

5. **Religious fasting:** Many religions have fasting practices, such as Ramadan fasting for Muslims, Yom Kippur fasting for Jews, and Lent fasting for Christians.

6. **Juice fasting:** This involves consuming only fruit and vegetable juices, and may be done for a few days to a few weeks.

7. **Modified fasting:** This involves consuming a limited number of calories or specific types of foods, such as vegetables, for a set period of time.

It's important to note that while fasting can have potential health benefits, it may not be suitable for everyone, especially individuals with certain medical conditions or nutrient deficiencies. It's important to consult a healthcare professional before attempting any form of fasting.

Fasting in different religions

Yom Kippur fasting

Yom Kippur is the holiest day of the Jewish year, and fasting is one of the central observances of the day. The fast begins at sundown on the eve of Yom Kippur and lasts until after nightfall the following day.

During this time, Jewish people refrain from eating, drinking, and engaging in other physical pleasures, as a way of atoning for sins and focusing on spiritual matters.

The practice of fasting on Yom Kippur is based on biblical commandments to "afflict your souls" and "deny yourselves" (Leviticus 16:29-31).

The idea is that by depriving oneself of physical needs, one can focus more fully on spiritual matters and on seeking forgiveness for one's sins.

Fasting on Yom Kippur is seen as a communal practice, with the entire Jewish community participating together in the fast. It is also a day of introspection and prayer, with services lasting throughout the day and focusing on themes of repentance and forgiveness.

However, there are some exceptions to the Yom Kippur fast, such as for individuals who are ill or pregnant, or for children under a certain age.

In these cases, it is considered more important to prioritize one's health and well-being over the observance of the fast.

Lent fasting

Lent is a Christian observance that involves a period of fasting, prayer, and repentance in the lead-up to Easter. The length of Lent varies depending on the denomination, but it typically lasts for around 40 days.

Fasting during Lent can take different forms, depending on the individual and their religious tradition.

Some Christians choose to give up a particular food or activity for the entire duration of Lent, as a form of sacrifice and discipline. Others may choose to fast on certain days of the week to abstain from meat on Fridays, in keeping with Catholic tradition.

The purpose of Lenten fasting is similar to that of Yom Kippur fasting, in that it is intended to help the individual focus on spiritual matters and prepare themselves for a holy occasion.

In the case of Lent, the focus is on the celebration of Easter, which commemorates the resurrection of Jesus Christ.

Fasting during Lent is often accompanied by other spiritual practices, such as prayer, charitable giving, and attending religious services.

The idea is to use this time to reflect on one's relationship with God, and to seek forgiveness for one's sins.

Again, there may be exceptions to the Lenten fast, particularly for individuals with health concerns.

Additionally, some Christian denominations may have specific guidelines or exemptions regarding fasting during Lent.

Fasting in Buddhism

Fasting in Buddhism is not as widely practiced as it is in other religions, such as Judaism or Christianity. However, there are some Buddhist traditions that involve fasting as a form of spiritual practice.

In Buddhist practice, fasting may be seen as a way to cultivate discipline and self-control, as well as to purify the body and mind. Fasting may also be undertaken as a form of penance or to atone for past misdeeds.

One form of Buddhist fasting is known as "uposatha," which involves abstaining from food and drink for a period of 24 hours, once or twice a month.

This practice is typically observed by monastics, but laypeople may also choose to observe it as a way of deepening their spiritual practice.

Another form of Buddhist fasting is known as "nyungne," which involves a more intense form of fasting and purification.

This practice is associated with the bodhisattva Avalokiteshvara and involves a two-day fasting retreat, during which participants abstain from food and drink for 24 hours, and then consume only one meal the following day. The practice is repeated for a total of two or three days, depending on the tradition.

In addition to these practices, there are also Buddhist traditions that involve periodic fasting or abstaining from certain foods or activities as a way of promoting spiritual growth and discipline.

However, fasting is generally viewed as a means to an end, rather than an end in itself, in Buddhist practice, with the ultimate goal being the attainment of enlightenment and liberation from suffering.

Fasting in Hinduism

Fasting is a common practice in Hinduism and is observed by millions of Hindus worldwide. Fasting, or "vrata," is considered a way to purify the body and mind, and to cultivate spiritual awareness and devotion to God.

There are many different forms of fasting in Hinduism, each with its own purpose and guidelines.

Hindu fasting may involve abstaining from food, water, or certain types of food for a specified period of time.

Some types of fasts may allow the consumption of certain foods or liquids, such as milk, fruit, or water. F

Fasting may be practiced individually or as a community and is often accompanied by prayer, meditation, and acts of charity.

The purpose of Hindu fasting is similar to that of fasting in other religions: to cultivate self-discipline, purify the body and mind, and deepen one's spiritual awareness and devotion to God.

Which days are forbidden to fast in Islam

In Islam, there are certain days when it is forbidden to fast. These include:

1. **Eid al-Fitr:** This is the festival that marks the end of the month of Ramadan. It is forbidden to fast on this day as it is a day of celebration and feasting.

2. **Eid al-Adha:** This is the festival that marks the end of the annual pilgrimage to Mecca (Hajj). It is also a day of celebration and feasting, so fasting is forbidden on this day as well.

3. **The three days of Tashreeq:** These are the 11th, 12th, and 13th days of the Islamic month of Dhul-Hijjah, which immediately follow the day of sacrifice (Eid al-Adha). It is forbidden to fast on these days.

4. **The day of Arafat:** This is the 9th day of the Islamic month of Dhul-Hijjah, which is the day before Eid al-Adha. It is recommended to fast on this day for those who are not performing the

pilgrimage, but it is forbidden for those who are performing the pilgrimage.

5. **The day of Ashura:** This is the 10th day of the Islamic month of Muharram. It is recommended to fast on this day, but it is not forbidden to eat or drink if one chooses not to fast.

6. **Fridays:** It is also forbidden to single out Fridays and only fast every Friday, as 'Abdullah B 'Amr b. al-'As said that he heard Muhammad say "Verily, Friday is an Eid (holiday) for you, so do not fast on it unless you fast the day before or after it."

7. **Fasting every day of the year:** is considered non-rewarding; Muhammad said: "There is no reward for fasting for the one who perpetually fasts." This Hadith is considered authentic by Sunni scholars.

It is important to note that these are the only days on which fasting is forbidden in Islam. Muslims are encouraged to fast voluntarily throughout the year, outside of the month of

Ramadan, as a way of increasing their spirituality and drawing closer to God.

Chapter 12

Ramadan and new convert Muslims

Ramadan is an important time for all Muslims, including new converts to Islam.

Here are some suggestions for how new converts can approach Ramadan:

1. **Learn about the significance of Ramadan:** New converts should learn about the importance and significance of Ramadan in Islam. They can do this by reading books, attending lectures, and speaking with other Muslims.

2. **Set achievable goals:** New converts should set achievable goals for themselves during Ramadan, such as reading Quran or attending taraweeh (nightly prayers during Ramadan) at the mosque.

3. **Seek support from the Muslim community:** New converts can seek support from the Muslim community during Ramadan. They can attend iftar (the meal that breaks the fast) at the

mosque, participate in group prayers, and seek advice and guidance from more experienced Muslims.

4. **Take care of their health:** New converts should take care of their health during Ramadan, mainly if they are not used to fasting. They should stay hydrated and avoid overeating during Iftar.

5. **Reflect on their journey to Islam:** Ramadan is a time for reflection and self-improvement. New converts can use this time to reflect on their journey to Islam and make plans for their future as Muslims.

Ramadan can be a challenging but rewarding time for new converts to Islam. They can approach it by learning about its significance, setting achievable goals, seeking support from the Muslim community, taking care of their health, and reflecting on their journey to Islam.

Testimonial from convert Muslims about Ramadan

Many converts to Islam find Ramadan to be a transformative and spiritually enriching experience. The month of fasting allows them to reflect on their faith and deepen their connection to Allah.

It provides an opportunity to detach from worldly distractions and focus on what truly matters. By abstaining from food and drink, as well as other permissible pleasures, they develop greater discipline and self-control.

Ramadan also fosters a sense of community among Muslims. Converts often feel a strong sense of belonging during this time as they come together with their fellow Muslims to break their fasts and perform nightly prayers.

It is a time of sharing, generosity, and kindness, which can be especially meaningful for converts who may have felt isolated before embracing Islam.

Many converts to Islam find Ramadan to be a transformative and deeply rewarding experience. It allows them to deepen their faith, connect with their community, and become better versions of themselves.

Testimonials:

1. Lovii Hicks said she recently found her religious calling. Her upbringing was Bible based. She grew up a Jehovah's Witness, became Catholic, and then practiced another Christian faith, but always felt something was missing.

   "Religion shouldn't be religious, it should be a spiritual connection," said Hicks. "You should have a direct line to your creator, and I didn't have that connection."

   Her thirst for knowledge and a desire for worship led her to Islam. She became Muslim in September 2021.

   "It means everything to me," said Hicks. "It gives me peace, and it centers me. Just taking those few 10 minutes out to pray five times a day is a blessing."

   Ramadan, which began in April, is her first. The holy month is an annual celebration for Muslims around the world. From sunrise to sunset, able-bodied Muslims are encouraged to abstain from eating and drinking as much as a sip of water.

"I thought it was going to be hard," said Hicks. "I was so scared. Like, I prepped, my house is Ramadan-proof now. I put all my snacks away. I don't have anything laying out that I could just reach and grab."

To the outside world, the month may seem like misery, but to the Muslim community, it's magical.

"It's not like you're sacrificing yourself, you're starving, you're walking around all gaunt and hungry," said Hicks. "You're full of worship and prayer and God's word that sustains you throughout the day. And then when it is time to eat, it's a feast."

2. Matt Schoonover became Muslim in 2006. Like Hicks, he didn't have a faith that resonated with him until he found Islam.

Ramadan comes at a different time every year because it is the ninth month of the Islamic calendar. Schoonover said his first Ramadan was difficult.

"The first Ramadan, it was more of a struggle for a couple of reasons. One, never being used to fasting before and then also, you know, 16 years ago, it was kind of more towards the summertime," said Schoonover.

"So it was starting, like the fasts were really, really long. So that makes it more difficult when you're fasting for, like 15, 16 hours as opposed to right now where it's 14 hours."

Ramadan is a reset for many Muslims. It's a time to take a step back, reflect and grow.

Muslims are encouraged to read the Quran and get to know more about their religion as well as themselves. It's not just about abstaining from food and water but abstaining from destructive behavior or character as well.

"[It] allows me to take time to reflect, you know, make myself a better Muslim, a better person, get rid of your bad deeds," said Schoonover. "It's definitely got me on the right track in terms of doing better deeds, for myself and for others."

3. I remember my first Ramadan like it was yesterday. It was the summer of 2015, and I was extremely new to the religion. I converted to Islam weeks before the holy month and had never fasted a day in my life even for medical reasons.

I am from a Catholic/Christian blended family who had no idea that I was even remotely interested in Islam. The next kicker is, I worked for my family's company that summer and I knew going into it that secretly fasting all day was going to be very difficult.

No one knew that I was converting to Islam, even my Muslim friends. I was so terrified of what everyone would say and think of me. Being a very sensitive person, I knew that if I were to face too much rejection, I would give up and continue trying to fit the square peg of Christianity into my circle heart.

I had very limited resources, as I only closely knew a handful of Muslims and had no idea if the information I was gathering was even accurate.

I was reading a book called "Introduction to Islam" along with the

Holy Quran and various website searches, desperate for anything that would help me. I did not have a support group, a family that took me in, or even a group of friends who could join me in this feat.

I live in the southern region of the United States so during the summer months, it gets very hot and near unbearable for someone who is new to fasting. I would sit at my desk and try to get through my work without water or food and read my books during lunch. When it was time to break my fast, I would just find something to eat outside alone and then go back home to prepare for the next day.

At this point in my life, I had no friends who lived close to me because I was home from College for the summer and was living and working with my family.

I did not make it through the entire month, but I thank Allah for that month of tests, trials, and self-realization.

Alhamdulilah for that time.

I just ask that everyone, no matter what stage you are in on your journey to

Islam, please remember those who have just entered the faith or are considering joining.

Pray that our new sisters and brothers who choose to fast will find it easy and will not give up.

Check on people who you know are struggling with fasting and invite them into your home for Iftar.

Keep communication open between friends this year who may need to lean on you a little.

As Prophet Muhammad (عليه السلام) once said: "Whoever helps his brother in his time of need, Allah will be there in his time of need"

I will leave you with this:

And as for those who strive in Our path — We will surely guide them in Our ways. And Indeed, Allah is with those who are of service to others. (Al Quran 29:70)

Conclusion and Reflections on Fasting

In conclusion, Ramadan fasting is a sacred and important practice in the Islamic faith. It is a time for spiritual reflection, prayer, and self-discipline.

Fasting during Ramadan helps to purify the mind and body, and provides an opportunity to connect with one's faith on a deeper level.

Throughout the month of Ramadan, Muslims fast from dawn to sunset, refraining from food, water, and other physical needs.

Fasting is not just about abstaining from food and drink, but also from negative thoughts, actions, and behaviors. It is a time to practice self-control, discipline, and patience.

Ramadan is also a time for increased prayer and spiritual reflection. Muslims are encouraged to read the Quran, attend Taraweeh prayers, and engage in other spiritual activities to strengthen their connection with Allah (SWT).

In addition to its spiritual benefits, Ramadan fasting has also been shown to have health benefits. Studies have shown that intermittent fasting can improve heart health, reduce inflammation, and promote weight loss.

Overall, Ramadan fasting is a beautiful and transformative practice that brings Muslims together in worship, prayer, and reflection. It is a time to renew one's faith, purify one's soul, and connect with the divine.

Ramadan is a significant month in the Islamic calendar that involves fasting, increased prayer, and acts of charity.

It is a time for self-reflection, spiritual growth, and strengthening one's relationship with Allah. Muslims believe that by abstaining from food and drink during daylight hours, they can develop greater self-discipline and empathy for those who are less fortunate.

Ramadan is also a time for increased social and communal activities, with families and friends gathering for Iftar (the breaking of the fast) and Suhoor (the pre-dawn meal).

Mosques are often filled with worshippers for Taraweeh prayers during the nights of Ramadan.

References

POORGIRLCHARMSCHOOL. (2019, May 5).
Ramadan: The True Testimony of a
Revert's Faith. *American Revert*.
Retrieved May 24, 2023, from
https://americanrevertdotcom.wordpress
.com/2019/05/05/ramadan-the-true-testi
mony-of-a-reverts-faith/

Kutty, S. A. K. (2022, April 1). Should the New
Moon for Ramadan Be Sighted or
Calculated? *About Islam*. Retrieved May
24, 2023, from
https://aboutislam.net/counseling/ask-th
e-scholar/fasting/should-the-new-moon-f
or-ramadan-be-sighted-or-calculated/

Cleveland, T. B. C. (2022, April 11). Observing
Ramadan through the eyes of new
Muslims. *Spectrum News1*. Retrieved
May 24, 2023, from
https://spectrumnews1.com/oh/columbu
s/news/2022/04/10/ramadan-through-th
e-eyes-of-new-muslims

Muslim hands. (2022, April 29). Special Edition
on ZAKAT UL-FITR and EID AL-FITR.
The Point. Retrieved May 24, 2023,

from
https://thepoint.gm/muslims-hands/speci
al-edition-on-special-edition-on-zakat-ul-
fitr-and-eid-al-fitr

Pilgrim. (2021). List of things that break your
fast. *Pilgrim*. Retrieved May 24, 2023,
from
https://thepilgrim.co/list-of-things-that-br
eak-your-fast/#:~:text=Things%20That%
20Don%27t%20Break,Swallowing%20y
our%20saliva

Soltani, A. S. (2022, March 30). Guide to
Understanding Ramadan. *Cair
Oklahoma*. Retrieved May 24, 2023,
from
https://www.cairoklahoma.com/blog/und
erstanding-ramadan/?gclid=Cj0KCQjw8
qmhBhCIARIsANAtboeSQmrPGzYebaT
WZoeezbK215S3snSlcatlBLa8lps2vFOj
dAKe4p0aAsjJEALw_wcB

Islam online. (2023). Ramadan and Quran.
Islam Online. Retrieved May 24, 2023,
from
https://islamonline.net/en/ramadan-and-t
he-quran/

watan UK. (2021). What is Zakat al-Fitr? *Watan UK*. Retrieved May 24, 2023, from https://www.watan.org.uk/religious-dues/zakat-al-fitr/#:~:text=The%20payment%20of%20Zakat%20al,who%20is%20dependent%20on%20you

Al Amanah. (2023). Prophet Noah. *Al Amanah College*. Retrieved May 24, 2023, from https://www.alamanah.nsw.edu.au/prophet-noah/#:~:text=Noah%20and%20Moses%20fasted%20that,Moses%20more%20than%20others%20do%20%E2%80%9D

NF studio. (2023). 6 Things Christians Should Know About Ramadan (and How to Support Muslims). *NF Studio*. Retrieved May 24, 2023, from https://www.neighborlyfaith.org/6-things-christians-should-know-about-ramadan?gclid=Cj0KCQjw8qmhBhCIARIsANAtboeR8hnZbK_nyOpeJDOVdsAPQppoeZ7MJN3c2vNDUQxvoD79anMbnD8aAkaZEALw_wcB#:~:text=WHAT%20THEY%20CELEBRATE.%22-,1.%20What%20Is%20Ramadan%3F,-Ramadan%20commemorates%20the

Srinagar news. (2023, March 21). Ramadan 2023 begins on March 23; crescent moon not sighted in Saudi Arabia. *Srinagar News*. Retrieved May 24, 2023, from https://srinagarnews.net/21/03/2023/ramadan-2023-begins-on-march-23-crescent-moon-not-sighted-in-saudi-arabia/

Spero, J. S. (2023, March 21). Ramadan: What to Know About the Muslim Holy Month in 2023. *Csun Today*. Retrieved May 24, 2023, from https://csunshinetoday.csun.edu/arts-and-culture/ramadan-what-to-know-about-the-muslim-holy-month-in-2023/

AlJazeera. (2023, March 23). Holy month of Ramadan begins for Muslims around the world. *AlJazeera*. Retrieved May 24, 2023, from https://www.aljazeera.com/gallery/2023/3/23/photos-holy-month-of-ramadan-begins-for-muslims-around-the-world

Dirgantoro, R. D. (2023, March 31). Fasting Benefits. *Shutterstock*. Retrieved May 25, 2023, from

https://www.shutterstock.com/image-vec
tor/intermittent-fasting-health-benefit-inf
o-graphic-1855476934

Freepik. (2010). Henna tattoo on woman hands
    artist drawing arabic mehndi. *Freepik*.
    Retrieved May 25, 2023, from
    https://www.freepik.com/premium-photo/
    henna-tattoo-woman-hands-artist-drawi
    ng-arabic-mehndi_17842331.htm

Hanafi, J. H. (2010). Chicken Biryani, Famoust
    Food of Pakistani & Indian People.
    Adobe Stock. Retrieved May 25, 2023,
    from
    https://stock.adobe.com/images/chicken
    -biryani-famoust-food-of-pakistani-indian
    -people/252459861

BreWoodsy. (2021, January 24). Samosa Food
    Snack. *Pixabay*. Retrieved May 25,
    2023, from
    https://pixabay.com/photos/samosa-food
    -snack-indian-fried-5936466/

Freepik. (2010a). Healthy fattoush salad.
    Freepik. Retrieved May 25, 2023, from
    https://www.freepik.com/premium-photo/
    healthy-fattoush-salad-closeup-key-ingr

edient-this-middle-eastern-dish-is-toasted-pita-bread-which-is-mixed-with-healthy-vegetables-herbs-dressing-made-with-lemon-sumac_30885963.htm

Freepik. (2010c). Traditional eastern desserts on wooden background. *Freepik*. Retrieved May 25, 2023, from https://www.freepik.com/free-photo/traditional-eastern-desserts-wooden-background_21064272.htm#query=turkish%20delight&position=0&from_view=keyword&track=ais

Platter of keboob. (2010). *Freepik*. Retrieved May 25, 2023, from https://www.freepik.com/premium-photo/platter-kebabs-uch-panzha-lamb-kebab-chicken-kebab-with-lamb-shish-kebab-chicken-lamb-skewers-plate-with-traditional-uzbekistan-ornament_13144797.htm